...heral Artery

"Peripheral artery disease frequently diminishes the quality of life of many older individuals. Patients with this problem receive care from their primary care physicians and specialists, including vascular surgeons, cardiologists, and interventional radiologists. Rarely do patients have an opportunity to see an expert vascular medicine specialist, like the authors, Drs. Mohler and Hirsch. Their passion for helping patients with this disease is evident in the introduction, and their expertise in the field is widely recognized. They are to be congratulated for creating this easy-to-read book that provides patients and their families with a comprehensive, up-to-date, and objective review of the most common aspects of peripheral artery disease."

Jon S. Matsumura, MD
Professor and Chief, Division of Vascular Surgery,
University of Wisconsin School of Medicine and Public Health

"This book is just what patients, their families, and their friends need: clear, concise information about a very serious and common medical problem. Peripheral artery disease is often overlooked, unrecognized, and poorly understood. Drs. Hirsch and Mohler, two experts in this area, are going to change this with their book."

John A. Kaufman, MD
Chief of Vascular and Interventional Radiology,
Dotter Interventional Institute
Frederick S. Keller Professor of Interventional Radiology,
Oregon Health & Science University Hospital
Portland, OR

D1082278

100 Questions & Answers About Peripheral Artery Disease (PAD)

Emile R. Mohler III, MD

*Director of Vascular Medicine
and Associate Professor of Medicine,
University of Pennsylvania Foundation
Philadelphia, PA*

Alan T. Hirsch, MD

*Director, Vascular Medicine Program
Minneapolis Heart Institute Foundation
at Abbott Northwestern Hospital
Minneapolis, MN*

JONES AND BARTLETT PUBLISHERS

Sudbury, Massachusetts

BOSTON   TORONTO   LONDON   SINGAPORE

World Headquarters

Jones and Bartlett Publishers	Jones and Bartlett Publishers	Jones and Bartlett Publishers
40 Tall Pine Drive	Canada	International
Sudbury, MA 01776	6339 Ormindale Way	Barb House, Barb Mews
978-443-5000	Mississauga, Ontario L5V 1J2	London W6 7PA
info@jbpub.com	Canada	United Kingdom
www.jbpub.com		

Jones and Bartlett's books and products are available through most bookstores and online book-sellers. To contact Jones and Bartlett Publishers directly, call 800-832-0034, fax 978-443-8000, or visit our website, www.jbpub.com.

Substantial discounts on bulk quantities of Jones and Bartlett's publications are available to corporations, professional associations, and other qualified organizations. For details and specific discount information, contact the special sales department at Jones and Bartlett via the above contact information or send an email to specialsales@jbpub.com

The authors, editor, and publisher have made every effort to provide accurate information. However, they are not responsible for errors, omissions, or for any outcomes related to the use of the contents of this book and take no responsibility for the use of the products and procedures described. Treatments and side effects described in this book may not be applicable to all people; likewise, some people may require a dose or experience a side effect that is not described herein. Drugs and medical devices are discussed that may have limited availability controlled by the Food and Drug Administration (FDA) for use only in a research study or clinical trial. Research, clinical practice, and government regulations often change the accepted standard in this field. When consideration is being given to use of any drug in the clinical setting, the healthcare provider or reader is responsible for determining FDA status of the drug, reading the package insert, and reviewing prescribing information for the most up-to-date recommendations on dose, precautions, and contraindications, and determining the appropriate usage for the product. This is especially important in the case of drugs that are new or seldom used.

Production Credits
Senior Acquisitions Editor: Alison Hankey
Editorial Assistant: Sara Cameron
Production Director: Amy Rose
Associate Production Editor: Jessica deMartin
Assistant Print Buyer: Jessica DeMarco
Composition: Glyph International
Printing and Binding: Malloy, Inc.

Cover Credits
Cover Design: Carolyn Downer
Cover Printing: Malloy, Inc.
Cover Images: Top left: © absolut/ShutterStock, Inc. Rights: Royalty Free; Bottom left: © Monkey Business Images/ShutterStock, Inc. Rights: Royalty Free; Right: © Monkey Business Images/Shutter Stock, Inc. Rights: Royalty Free

Library of Congress Cataloging-in-Publication Data
Mohler, Emile R.
  100 questions & answers about peripheral artery disease (PAD) / Emile R. Mohler, III and Alan T. Hirsch.
    p. cm.
  Includes index.
  ISBN 978-0-7637-5866-0
  1. Peripheral vascular diseases—Miscellanea. I. Hirsch, Alan T. (Alan Tick) II. Title. III. Title: 100 questions and answers about peripheral artery disease (PSD). IV. Title: One hundred questions and answers about peripheral artery disease (PSD).
  RC694.M64 2010
  616.1'31—dc22
                                          2009025874
6048
Printed in the United States of America
13 12 11 10 09   10 9 8 7 6 5 4 3 2 1

This book is dedicated to:

The Hirsch family:
Jonathan and Rebecca;
Margot, Bob, and Jan; Gail and Bill;
Brent and Yael; and Leigh and Jeremy,
and to those others who know they are loved;

and to:

The Mohler family

Life lessons and love:

In dedication to Robert L. David, 1916–1988

Robert David was a loving husband and father to four. Born in Rochester, NY in 1916, he graduated from the University of Michigan before joining the Army Air Force and serving in the Pacific theater during World War II. After the war ended he married the love of his life, Joan, and settled down to raise his family, manage his business, and support his community in suburban Chicago. He was an avid golfer and a top-level bridge player who had a voracious appetite for living life to the fullest.

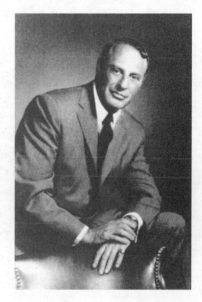

Unfortunately, like many individuals before and after the War, Bob began smoking at an early age. The combination of his addiction to nicotine, which he never overcame, and a family history of high cholesterol led to a life-long struggle with arterial disease. After years of enduring leg pain when he walked, and finally obtaining a PAD diagnosis, he underwent leg bypass surgery in 1976. At the time, leg angioplasty, claudication medications, and most preventative therapies were not available. Bob subsequently suffered two heart attacks, with debilitating impacts on his life and family. Thereafter, he underwent heart bypass surgery in 1981 and an additional major surgical procedure in 1983 to repair an abdominal aortic aneurysm. Bob's PAD led to the loss of one leg in 1984, and the loss of his second leg in 1986, on his 70th birthday. Despite his illness, his joy for life, family, and friends remained keen. He passed away in 1988.

Bob's illness began long before much was known about peripheral artery disease. These were times that were well before doctors routinely prescribed statins for patients with high cholesterol, provided tobacco cessation therapies for those who smoked, or before many vascular specialists, primary care physicians, and nurses had acquired the expertise to detect PAD early to prevent its progression or its complications. Unfortunately, we are aware that many individuals and families, despite 20 years of medical advances, continue to be deprived of access to effective care, and thus to hope.

Too many lives have been lost to PAD. Wives need their husbands; husbands need their wives; children need their parents. Bob knew these facts well, and would be pleased if you would heed his joy for life. Take care to prevent PAD, treat it promptly, and enjoy the gift of life.

— The Family of Robert L. David

Contents

Part 1: Peripheral Artery Disease (PAD) Epidemiology and Prevalence   1

Questions 1–9 introduce important, basic facts about PAD, including:
- How common is PAD?
- Can PAD be prevented or cured?
- Does PAD affect some ethnic groups more than others?

Part 2: PAD Pathophysiology   9

Questions 10–20 describe some of the ways PAD affects the body, such as:
- What causes a blocked artery in the leg?
- Can the artery in my leg suddenly clot off?
- What causes gangrene of the foot?

Part 3: Symptoms and Physical Findings of PAD   17

Questions 21–30 review the common symptoms associated with PAD, like:
- What is claudication?
- What is a foot ulcer and can it be caused by PAD?
- Can the arteries in my arms get blockages like those in leg arteries and cause pain?

Part 4: PAD Diagnosis   25

Questions 31–41 provide an overview of how PAD is diagnosed, including:
- What is an ankle-brachial index (ABI) test?
- What is a duplex arterial ultrasound?
- What is a catheter angiogram?

Contents

If you are like most people, then you value being able to grow through adolescence into adulthood, to find a life partner, and then to live with personal independence, yet close to those you love. You also likely want to sustain this freedom throughout your older years. This desire to enjoy one's life and to participate in the lives of one's children and grandchildren is universal. Yet, as we navigate through life, many illnesses can deprive us of this joy. One of the most common and potentially dangerous (although easily treated) of these illnesses is peripheral artery disease, also known simply as PAD.

What? You'd never heard of PAD until recently? If so, then you are like the tens of millions of individuals throughout the world who simply have never been provided easy access to information about this common disease.

Why should you, and all adults throughout the world, know about PAD? Very simply because without this knowledge, you cannot protect yourself and your loved ones in order to achieve the dreams that define your life.

When you exercise, your muscles work to propel your body forward to help you achieve your immediate goal, on a journey to accomplish your long-term dreams. Half your body (your legs) is devoted to this mission, permitting your mind to propel you through the world so your hands can work or reach out to embrace those you love. As you work, your heart will beat stronger and your lungs will breathe deeper. Together, your heart and lungs will deliver the oxygen and nutrients needed by your leg muscles as they seek to work harder.

In some people, however, atherosclerosis (hardening of the arteries) restricts this blood flow. When your muscles don't get the oxygen and nutrients they need during exercise, such as walking, you experience a cramping discomfort called claudication. This symptom is sometimes called "intermittent" claudication because the pain stops with rest.

This muscle fatigue, discomfort, or pain is one of the primary symptoms of PAD, a disease of the arteries beyond the heart. It typically affects the blood supply to the legs and results from clogged arteries. It is usually a sign that there is atherosclerotic disease elsewhere in the body, such as the brain, heart, or kidneys.

Unfortunately, you can have this dangerous condition even if you don't have any symptoms. Many people don't experience any muscle discomfort or intermittent claudication until the artery is blocked or occluded by 60% or more. Thus, during the years or even decades while PAD is developing, you may be unaware of what is happening inside your arteries. Even when you start to experience some symptoms, you may just assume these aches and pains in your leg muscles are a natural part of getting old.

However, when arteries are damaged by atherosclerosis in one site (such as the leg arteries), they are likely also damaged in other vital locations (such as the heart or brain). If a blood clot forms in a damaged artery to the heart or brain, a narrowed, diseased artery can suddenly close off completely, leading to a heart attack or stroke. That is why people with PAD have an increased risk for both of these conditions. In fact, the risk of dying from heart disease is six to seven times higher in those with PAD compared to those without.

We know from our experience, and from the scientific studies completed by so many of our hard-working colleagues, that you can survive and thrive with PAD. This book is intended to offer you the information you need to do this and the information your family needs to help you. This book is also intended to offer you the inspiration and hope you deserve to be successful.

If you achieve your dreams, we will have achieved ours.

With the strength of our convictions and our belief in yours,

Emile R. Mohler III, MD
Alan T. Hirsch, MD

Why a Book for Patients About PAD? Five Perspectives

It has been challenging for individuals with vascular diseases to obtain reliable, accurate information. Moreover, because care for peripheral artery disease, known as PAD, throughout the world is often provided by both primary care and vascular specialty physicians with widely differing training, patients and families can become confused by conflicting perspectives. We therefore begin this book by providing the views of each of these kinds of physicians, who represent the very best of their field of training. Views are shared from an internal medicine physician/vascular medicine specialist, a vascular surgeon, an interventional radiologist, and a primary care internist. We also acknowledge that empowerment of patients and aid in considering care decisions are often best accomplished with the help of an experienced vascular nurse. We hope that these perspectives also help you. Our goal is to ensure that when you consider bringing such questions to your own physicians, you will be confident that we have provided a genuinely interdisciplinary perspective.

Alan T. Hirsch and Emile R. Mohler III

Why Should You Care About Peripheral Artery Disease?

Perspective 1: The internist and vascular medicine specialist

I'm delighted to introduce this book dedicated to informing the public about the importance of peripheral artery disease. This is a disorder closely related to heart disease and stroke but is often missed by physicians and patients alike. When unrecognized, it can lead to deleterious consequences. If we think in the broadest terms, diseases of the arteries (atherosclerosis, or hardening of the arteries) create the greatest health burden for our society. We are all quite familiar with the risks of heart attack and stroke that can lead to premature death; or in those who survive, there is the burden of tremendous physical limitations. Peripheral artery disease has a similar fate, but it mainly involves the legs and leads to a drastic reduction in the ability to walk and to perform daily activities. But more importantly, as a disease of all blood vessels, peripheral artery disease is highly related to the risk of stroke and heart attack, and still more importantly, these risks can be prevented with proper therapies. Therefore, as a vascular medicine specialist, I work hard with my patients to control their risk factors for heart disease and stroke as well as provide therapies to treat the symptoms in their legs.

One of the important missions of our vascular community, including the Vascular Disease Foundation and the PAD Coalition, is to expand public awareness of peripheral artery disease. We have discovered from previous studies that over half the individuals with this disorder are unaware of it, even though they may have symptoms in their legs or struggle to complete their daily activities, all of which could be related to PAD. We hope that with simple diagnostic tests commonly available in doctors' offices and the broader community, we will be able to detect this disease early and therefore prevent the severe consequences of the disorder. This book is one of those steps forward in building awareness and improving treatment and outcomes in peripheral artery disease.

William R. Hiatt, MD
Professor of Medicine
University of Colorado, School of Medicine
President, Colorado Prevention Center
Denver, CO

Perspective 2: The vascular surgeon

This book contains vital information you need to know about your blood vessels. Coauthored by two expert vascular physicians,

Drs. Mohler and Hirsch, the book provides easy-to-understand answers to 100 key questions about PAD.

Most patients with PAD have poor circulation in their legs due to hardening and narrowing of the arteries. The disease can also affect the aorta or other arteries that go to the brain, the arms, the kidneys, or the stomach. Read this book to find out causes and risk factors of PAD and presenting symptoms such as pain when walking and resting, sores, and ulcers. Learn what the risk of losing a limb from PAD really is and about evaluation and management of this important disease. Look for questions and answers on prevention and on how to prolong your life with exercise and diet and with modifying other risk factors such as smoking, diabetes, or hypertension. There are questions and answers on medications and on minimally invasive new endovascular therapies, such as angioplasty or stents. Finally, learn why open surgery is effective and durable to salvage your affected limb.

Vascular specialists, including vascular and endovascular surgeons, have made tremendous progress in recent years in fighting PAD, and this book reflects the most recent changes. The authors and their public organizations, the PAD Coalition and the Vascular Disease Foundation, should be congratulated for their noble efforts to increase public awareness of PAD and for saving limbs and lives of patients affected by PAD.

Peter Gloviczki, MD
John M. and Ruth Roberts Professor of Surgery
Chair, Division of Vascular and Endovascular Surgery
Director, Gonda Vascular Center
Mayo Clinic
Rochester, MN

Perspective 3: The interventional radiologist

Peripheral artery disease currently afflicts over 9 million Americans. It can be disabling, can lead to poor quality of life, and is associated with increased risk of heart attacks, strokes, and death. For a disease that is so prevalent and associated with significant increased risk and decreased quality of life, it is poorly understood. Many healthcare professionals and lay people underestimate its importance.

It is a pleasure to be invited to write an introduction to this book from the perspective of an interventional radiologist, the specialty of medicine that developed catheter-based minimally invasive X-ray–guided treatment for artery blockages such as angioplasty and stent placement. While interventions such as angioplasty and stent placement can technically be done for many artery blockages, they, in fact, offer little benefit to patients in many cases, and noninvasive treatments are often preferred.

There are few clinicians and researchers such as Drs. Mohler and Hirsch with the extensive knowledge of vascular disease and the understanding of the individual and public health considerations that are needed for a book such as this. They are to be commended for their ability to clear the air on this topic. In their usual brilliant and lucid style, they have pulled together all of the necessary details in a clear and concise manner. In terms that can be understood by all, they describe what is known about PAD and what knowledge gaps need to be filled, and, in particular, they outline when invasive procedures are warranted and when they may be unnecessary. As an interventional radiologist, I am pleased to see this information presented to the public so they can make informed healthcare decisions. This volume is an indispensible addition to the library of anyone with an interest on the important topic of PAD.

Timothy P. Murphy, MD

Professor of Radiology, Brown University
Director, Department of Diagnostic Imaging
Medical Director, Rhode Island Hospital Vascular Disease Research Center
Rhode Island Hospital
Providence, RI

Perspective 4: The primary care internist

The primary care physician is frequently the first caregiver to suspect and diagnose PAD, a blood vessel disease that affects the legs and, to a lesser extent, the arms. As many as one out of five adults over the age of 65 may have PAD. Studies show that this disease is not limited to older men; women are equally at risk to develop PAD. Patients with PAD very often have other vascular diseases including coronary artery disease (involving blood vessels to the heart) and cerebrovascular disease (involving blood vessels to the brain) that can lead to heart attack and stroke. What is most alarming is that more than half of patients with PAD, both in North America and worldwide, are without symptoms and therefore are not taking appropriate measures to prevent the devastating consequences of this disease. The good news is that this condition can be easily diagnosed, and patients with PAD can take an active role in halting and even reversing the disease process.

This unique book, *100 Questions & Answers About Peripheral Artery Disease (PAD),* makes use of a question-and-answer format to address important issues related to PAD. The contents cover all aspects of PAD, and the organization allows you to read from cover to cover for a comprehensive review of the "most important disease no one has ever heard of" or to read just on the topics that are most pertinent to you. This book, with its patient-centered approach, will allow you to work hand-in-hand with your primary care doctor and vascular specialist to care for this condition. Most importantly, this book will empower you with useful, up-to-date, and detailed information to take an active role in your health care as it relates to PAD and to ensure the best possible care and health outcomes.

Patrick C. Alguire, MD, FACP
Director, Education and Career Development
American College of Physicians
Philadelphia, PA

Foreword

Perspective 5: The vascular nurse

I am so excited to be able to introduce this new resource for the public about peripheral artery disease. As a vascular nurse, clinician, and researcher, I am devoted to increasing awareness and improving the lives of those with this very important, but often unrecognized, disease. PAD is a common disease, caused by the build-up of fatty deposits in the arteries of the legs. This process is very similar to the build-up that causes decreased blood flow to the heart and the brain, causing heart attacks and strokes. In fact, individuals who have PAD are at very high risk of having a heart attack or stroke, even if they don't know they have the disease.

PAD causes a symptom called claudication, which is pain or discomfort caused by decreased blood supply to the leg muscles during physical activity. Claudication can make it difficult to walk even short distances without pain. We know from talking with our patients that this pain interferes with their ability to do the things they wish to do and can lead to significant disability and decreased quality of life.

One of the biggest problems with PAD is the lack of awareness about this debilitating and often dangerous disease among both the public and healthcare professionals. Too often, people think that leg pain when walking is a "normal" part of aging and is not important enough to complain about to their healthcare providers. Since PAD most often affects older adults, the claudication pain they experience is often thought to be caused by arthritis, joint problems, or back problems, when it is actually caused by decreased blood flow to the leg muscles. Having leg pain with aging is not normal and can only be effectively treated when the cause is correctly identified. Sometimes, even after being told they have PAD, patients are told that nothing can be done or that this isn't a dangerous disease. Some are told that they just have to live with their pain—that while it is uncomfortable, it isn't dangerous. Neither of these statements is true.

This book will make great strides in increasing public awareness of PAD. It will serve as a resource, dispelling myths and misinformation and providing up-to-date, accurate information based on our best knowledge about PAD. It will help people understand what PAD is, who is at risk, and what should be done after a diagnosis is made. I hope that resources such as this will help to improve the lives of patients with PAD, encouraging them to seek help sooner, decreasing their risk of disability and death, and improving the quality of their lives.

Diane Treat-Jacobson, PhD, RN, FAHA
Associate Professor of Nursing
University of Minnesota School of Nursing
Minneapolis, MN
Past-President, Society for Vascular Nursing

I am a 60-year-old married college professor with two grown children and three grandchildren.

As I think back, approximately two years ago I began to have mild discomfort in my left calf. I should have known and reacted sooner when the discomfort became cramping and pain when walking, but I told myself it was probably some sort of injury that was simply taking time to "work itself out." Additionally, I had breast cancer surgery in 2001, which is still medically monitored, and lung surgery in 2003. I was frankly tired of going to the doctor and therefore put off seeking medical assistance for my leg.

When I could not walk one block without pain, I realized that it was time to do something. I researched, found, and made an appointment with an excellent vascular cardiologist. After testing, I was diagnosed with PAD and it was discovered that I had 95% occlusion in the iliac artery of my left leg. I was fortunate in that a stent placement was an option and after the procedure, I was able to walk again without pain.

I know that my PAD is not cured but I also know that if I adhere to a medication maintenance, diet, and exercise plan, I can hope to prevent future blockages.

Mary Zaccagnini, DNP, RN, ACNS-BC, AOCN
Clinical Assistant Professor
University of Minnesota, School of Nursing
Minneapolis, MN

Acknowledgment

Life is precious, protecting life is a sacred mission, and inspiring hope is an act of love. We learned these lessons from our family and friends, we live with these thoughts each day, and we leave this vision as a legacy for our children. We now share our knowledge with you, anticipating that you will live each day in health.

PART ONE

Peripheral Artery Disease (PAD) Epidemiology and Prevalence

How common is PAD?

Can PAD be prevented or cured?

Does PAD affect some ethnic groups more than others?

More . . .

Epidemiology is defined as the study of the causes, distribution, and control of diseases in populations. The medical field of epidemiology asks questions such as, "What factors lead to the development of PAD?" "Why do certain people develop PAD and others do not?" and "How can our community decrease the impact of PAD?"

Prevalence is a term that describes the proportion of individuals who have a particular disease, such as PAD, at a particular time. When we ask, "What is the prevalence of PAD in my region?" we are asking for an estimate of how many people in our community right now have PAD, whether they know it or not.

Arteries

Blood vessels that carry blood away from the heart, supplying nutrition and oxygen to all of the tissues of the body.

Veins

Blood vessels that return blood from body tissue back to the heart.

Lymphatics

Microscopic vessels that transport fluid and protein from all of the tissues of the body, and that connect to the lymph glands. When these tiny vessels are blocked, swelling can occur that is called "lymphedema." This disease has no relationship to PAD.

Coronary arteries

The arteries that supply blood, oxygen, and nutrients to the heart.

Aorta

The major artery that leaves the heart and whose branches supply the rest of the body.

1. What is PAD?

Before we begin our discussion of this disease, it may be helpful to review the basic functions of the circulatory system. The blood vessels that leave the heart are called **arteries**, and the blood vessels that return blood to the heart are called **veins**. There are also microscopic vessels that carry fat and antibodies, which are called **lymphatics**.

Arteries supply nutrition and oxygen to all of the tissues of the body. The arteries that supply the heart are known as the **coronary arteries**, and these are "central." Thus, all of the other arteries are "peripheral," though they are just as critical to your health as the heart arteries. The major artery that leaves the heart is called the **aorta**. Other arteries include the carotid and vertebral arteries, which supply the brain; the subclavian, axillary, brachial, radial, and ulnar arteries, which supply the arms; the renal arteries, which supply the kidneys; and the celiac, superior mesenteric, and inferior mesenteric arteries, which supply the gut.

Peripheral artery disease (PAD) is defined as the broad group of disorders that affects any artery other than those that supply the heart itself. In most common usage, PAD implies disease of the arteries that supply the legs, as most recognized illness occurs in these vessels (**Figure 1**). Lower extremity PAD is most commonly caused by **atherosclerosis**, and refers to blockage of the inner lining of an artery by fatty deposits, resulting in poor perfusion of the skin, muscles, and limb.

Peripheral artery disease (PAD)

The broad group of disorders that affects any artery other than those that supply the heart itself. In most common usage, PAD implies disease of the arteries that supply the legs, as most recognized illness occurs in these vessels.

Atherosclerosis

A blockage of the inner lining of an artery by cholesterol deposits, resulting in poor blood flow to the skin, muscles, or other body organs. This disease, also known as "hardening of the arteries," is caused by smoking, diabetes, high blood pressure, elevated blood cholesterol, or inherited factors. Atherosclerosis is the most common cause of lower extremity PAD.

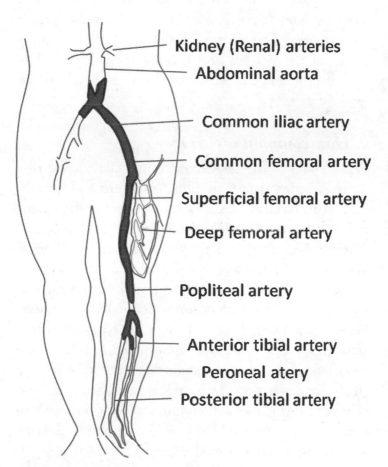

Kidney (Renal) arteries
Abdominal aorta
Common iliac artery
Common femoral artery
Superficial femoral artery
Deep femoral artery
Popliteal artery
Anterior tibial artery
Peroneal atery
Posterior tibial artery

Figure 1 The arteries most commonly affected by PAD. The shaded region depicts where cholesterol build up tends to occur.

Prior to 2000, many physicians would use the term "*peripheral vascular disease*" or "*PVD*" to describe the blockage in these leg arteries. Unfortunately, this term does not distinguish arteries from veins or lymphatic vessels, and thus it is confusing to both doctors and patients alike. Per USA and other international scientific statements, this older term should not be used anymore when referring to PAD.

As for any illness, patients who understand basic medical terms are likely to obtain better care. The term "P.A.D." is sometimes written with periods after each letter, in order to clarify for the public how this term is pronounced. Most doctors and other clinicians simply leave out the periods and use the term "PAD." The term is pronounced "pee-ay-dee" and not "pad," like a "pad" of paper.

PAD is one of the most common cardiovascular diseases, affecting over 9 million Americans and over 10 million Europeans.

2. How common is PAD?

PAD is one of the most common cardiovascular diseases, affecting over 9 million Americans and over 10 million Europeans. PAD is equally common in Central and South America, the Middle East, Asia, and Australia. As many as 1 in 20 adults over age 50 years and 1 in 4 adults over age 70 years are likely to be affected by PAD. This disease affects both men and women and is more common in individuals with **diabetes**, those who have a history of past or current smoking, and/or those who are exposed to other common atherosclerosis risk factors, such as hypertension (high blood pressure). Because these risk factors are also common, PAD is known to affect at least one adult in nearly every family. PAD is more common in African Americans. If you have PAD, you are not alone.

Diabetes

A condition where the body is unable to produce or use insulin properly, causing too high levels of sugar in the blood. Diabetes is one of the major risk factors for PAD.

3. Does PAD occur throughout the world?

There are no communities or nations that have avoided being affected by PAD. As noted in the previous question, PAD is common in North America, Central and South America, Europe and Russia, the Middle East, and China and Japan. This universally high prevalence is likely because PAD increases in *all* people as we age and also because citizens of every nation are exposed to common (and often avoidable) risk factors for artery disease. As individuals throughout the world increasingly gain weight, suffer from diabetes, smoke, and have high blood pressure and high blood cholesterol levels, PAD unfortunately becomes more common. PAD can be considered part of an "atherosclerosis pandemic." Newly developing nations can learn lessons from those who had no warning: By preventing these risk factors from affecting your citizens, PAD can be prevented.

4. Does PAD affect as many women as it does men?

Yes, PAD is equally common in women as in men (or perhaps even more common). Years ago, PAD was thought to be more common in men, but this is likely because the peak incidence of PAD occurs 5 to 10 years later in life in women. PAD rates rise steeply in women after menopause, but PAD can also occur in young women, especially those who smoke and/or have high blood cholesterol (PAD can also occur in young men). Since men have a shorter life span than women, more women ultimately survive to suffer from PAD.

High-sensitivity C-reactive protein (hs-CRP)

A protein that exists in the blood of all people and that increases in response to infection or inflammatory diseases (like some arthritis conditions). It is also increased in individuals with progressive atherosclerosis.

Thrombosis

The condition that occurs when blood clots develop in an artery.

Embolism

The condition that occurs when a blood clot travels from the heart to a more distant artery, blocking flow of blood.

Fibromuscular dysplasia

A condition, also known as FMD, due to abnormal growth of the arterial walls, which can cause a decrease in blood flow. When this occurs in the neck (carotid or vertebral) arteries, a stroke may occur. When this occurs in the arteries to the kidneys, hypertension may occur.

Thromboangiitis obliterans

A relatively rare disease, also called Buerger's disease, that is associated with inflammation and clotting of the arteries beyond the elbows and knees. It is more common in young men who use tobacco, though its cause is unknown.

5. Who is at risk of PAD?

As noted in Questions 2 through 4, PAD usually does not occur simply in response to aging. While age is a risk factor for PAD, artery blockage also occurs much more frequently and rapidly in individuals whose arteries are actively damaged by any of the following:

- Exposure to tobacco in any form (whether smoked or chewed)
- Diabetes (whether type I or type 2)
- High blood pressure (blood pressures higher than 140/80 mm Hg in most people, or greater than 130/80 mm Hg in individuals with diabetes)
- High blood cholesterol (usually defined as a total cholesterol greater than 200 mg/dL or a low-density lipoprotein [LDL] cholesterol level greater than 130 mg/dL)
- High levels of **high-sensitivity C-reactive protein** (sometimes abbreviated as hs-CRP)

For more information on each of these risk factors, see Questions 43–49.

Finally, individuals are at risk of having PAD if they have artery disease anywhere in their body, such as in the coronary (as in people who have suffered a prior heart attack, or undergone coronary angioplasty or bypass surgery) or carotid arteries (as in people who have suffered a prior stroke, or undergone carotid artery endarterectomy or angioplasty), or if they have an aortic aneurysm (or have undergone prior aortic aneurysm repair).

Mary's comment:

Although I had been diagnosed with high cholesterol and have a family history of cardiovascular disease, I was shocked to be diagnosed with PAD. I do not have high blood pressure nor diabetes, I do not smoke, and I am being treated for high cholesterol. In addition, I had only been aware of this diagnosis being given to people over 65 years old, which I am not. This just demonstrates that everyone should be aware of the symptoms of PAD, and should report them to their physician if discovered.

6. What are the less common causes of PAD?

PAD can also be caused, much less frequently, by other illnesses that can lead to artery blockage. Such illnesses can occur when clots develop in the artery itself (**thrombosis**) or when clots travel from the heart to a more distant artery (**embolism**). Other diseases that can block leg arteries include **fibromuscular dysplasia, thromboangiitis obliterans** (also called Buerger's disease), **popliteal adventitial cysts**, **arterial entrapment syndrome**, **large vessel arteritis** (inflammation of blood vessel), as well as other even rarer disorders. The term PAD also is sometimes used to include the diseases that cause a ballooning (**aneurysm**) of the aorta or other arteries. In this book, as in most medical practices, we will only discuss the impact of diseases that narrow the arteries.

7. Can PAD be prevented or cured?

PAD can be prevented by assuring that you minimize or eliminate your exposure to PAD risk factors. For example, *any* tobacco exposure at all (even from other people who smoke in your presence) is extremely damaging. Once artery damage starts, it is hard to prevent it from worsening. And, once present, it cannot be reversed or "fixed," not even by **angioplasty**, insertion of a metal **stent**, or surgery. There is no medication that can reverse existing damage. Knowing this, prevent PAD from starting and prevent PAD from worsening!

Popliteal adventitial cysts

The popliteal artery can in rare cases be blocked by "cystic adventitial disease." These cysts develop between the middle and outer layers of the wall of this knee artery. The cause of these cysts is unknown, could be hereditary or due to repetitive artery trauma. Such cysts occur more frequently in young men with new onset of claudication.

Arterial entrapment syndrome

A rare condition where arteries (which must often travel between muscle groups, or between muscles and bones, in order to reach the arms and legs) become briefly blocked or "entrapped" during very vigorous exercise. This can sometimes be an unusual cause of claudication.

Large vessel arteritis

Rather rarely, arteries can be damaged by diseases that cause inflammation of the artery wall. These diseases are treated very differently than when arteries are affected by atherosclerosis.

Aneurysm

An expansion or "ballooning" of the aorta or other arteries. Not all aneurysms are dangerous, but all should be followed by your doctor to verify if they are expanding.

Angioplasty

A procedure that opens clogged arteries by compressing obstructing plaque against the artery wall by inflation of a small balloon that is on the tip of the catheter.

Stent

A tubular metal device that is implanted into a blocked artery to hold it open and allow freer flow of blood.

There is no medication that can reverse existing damage. Knowing this, prevent PAD from starting and prevent PAD from worsening!

If you have PAD, the fact is that you will have PAD for the rest of your life. But, you can succeed in sustaining your health, protecting your life, and maintaining your independence by seeking good care and caring for yourself.

8. Does PAD affect some ethnic groups more than others?

Yes. Although PAD can affect anyone—men and women, young and old—it is more common in individuals of African American descent, who are at approximately a two-fold increased risk for PAD that is not explained by other risk factors nor other socioeconomic factors (such as income, work, or geography). The reasons for this increased risk remain unknown. Also, in North America it is known that Native Americans are also at increased risk, though this could be due to their much higher incidence of obesity and diabetes.

9. At what age does PAD most commonly occur?

As noted above, PAD is more common in individuals who are over 50 years of age. PAD becomes progressively more common with each decade of life. Almost one in four individuals over age 70 years have PAD.

PART TWO

PAD
Pathophysiology

What causes a blocked artery in the leg?

Can the artery in my leg suddenly clot off?

What causes gangrene of the foot?

More . . .

Physiology *is the study of the mechanisms that permit the body to function normally and usually relies on intricate mechanisms that maintain good health.* Pathophysiology *describes the abnormalities of function that occur when a part of the body no longer works normally. For individuals with PAD, the arteries may be moderately or severely blocked, and this can lead to abnormal blood flow, development of symptoms, clots, or the death of tissue downstream. The process by which damage to a healthy vessel leads to notable abnormalities of limb function is described as the "pathophysiology of PAD." Exploration of this pathophysiology helps us understand the consequences of the disease and how treatments might work to sustain health.*

10. What is the anatomy of leg arteries?

The aorta, the large blood vessel originating from the heart, divides into a right and left artery at the level of the umbilicus (belly button). These two main vessels are known as the iliac arteries (see Figure 1 in Question 1). The iliac artery continues into the leg, where it is referred to as the common femoral artery. The common femoral artery then divides into the superficial femoral artery and the deep femoral artery in order to supply the muscles of the thigh and the remainder of the leg. At the level of the knee, the superficial femoral artery becomes the popliteal artery. The popliteal artery divides into three major blood vessels that continue down the leg below the knee: the anterior tibial artery, the posterior tibial artery, and the peroneal artery.

11. What causes a blocked artery in the leg?

PAD can be caused by a large number of diseases that can either block or expand the arteries outside the heart. Most commonly, PAD is caused when the arteries to the legs become narrowed or clogged with cholesterol deposits, or **plaque** (pronounced "plak").

The buildup of plaque causes the arteries to harden and narrow, which is called atherosclerosis (pronounced "ath-uh-ro-skluh-RO-siss") (**Figure 2**). When leg arteries are hardened and clogged, blood flow to the legs and feet is reduced.

The most common cause of a blocked leg artery is buildup of cholesterol into a plaque that may protrude into the bloodstream, causing reduced blood flow. Other rare causes of a blocked leg artery include compression of an abnormal popliteal artery from adjacent muscle (known as popliteal entrapment) or compression from a cyst that is attached to the artery wall (known as adventitial cystic disease). Another relatively rare cause of a blocked leg artery is a blood clot that travels from the heart to lodge downstream in a small leg artery.

> **Plaque**
>
> Fatty deposits that narrow or clog arteries and can cause PAD.

PAD Pathophysiology

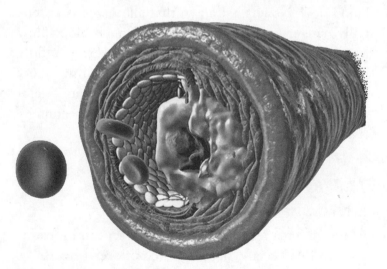

Figure 2   An example of how the inside of an atherosclerotic artery looks. (Courtesty Exploria Productions, LLC.)

12. What is plaque in the leg arteries made of?

Plaque is composed of variable quantities of cholesterol, fibrous tissue (scar tissue), white cells, and calcium.

Plaque is not the same in every artery or in every individual. Plaques can be variably obstructive (projecting into the artery and blocking blood flow), or they can be smaller and more fragile (even small amounts of plaque mean major damage has been done). Sometimes plaque has a hard lining that protects the inner substances of the plaque from exposure to the blood. These plaques are less dangerous, as they more rarely rupture and cause a clot to form in the artery. Other plaques have a thin and fragile lining that can break suddenly and unpredictably, causing a clot to form. Such clots are the cause of most heart attacks and many strokes.

All plaque is potentially dangerous, regardless of how much blood flow is obstructed.

Until the mid-1990s, it was thought that the most dangerous plaques were those most obstructive to blood flow. Now it is known that all plaque is potentially dangerous, regardless of how much blood flow is obstructed. Thus, a person can have mildly obstructive plaque and feel perfectly healthy. Then, suddenly the plaque lining may break, forming a clot that causes a heart attack, stroke, or death seemingly "without warning."

13. Why do my leg muscles hurt when exercising?

Although leg artery blockages are present in individuals with PAD even when they are not exercising, these blockages do not hurt because the legs do not require much blood supply when at rest. However, when you begin to perform any exercise, the work of moving your body requires a major (up to 30-fold) increase in leg muscle blood flow. Thus, with exercise, one or more blockages in the leg arteries may reduce blood flow to the leg muscles to the point where there is a major limitation of delivery of blood, nutrients, and oxygen to these working muscles. The response of the leg muscle to such a major reduction in oxygen is discomfort, or **claudication** (see Question 22).

Mary's comment:

I decided to see my doctor when I realized I could not walk on my treadmill for more than five minutes without muscle pain, and I had to rest due to pain occurring after I had walked only one block in my attempt to walk three blocks to meet my students for lunch. I was diagnosed with claudicaion and it was discovered that the iliac artery supplying my left leg was 93% blocked.

14. Can the artery in my leg suddenly clot off?

Yes. A sudden and complete occlusion of the artery in the leg is called **acute arterial occlusion** or acute limb ischemia, which is sometimes abbreviated ALI. This condition is, however, a relatively rare phenomenon and typically occurs due to either a blood clot (thrombus) traveling from upstream (the heart) or an aortic or popliteal aneurysm to a more distant leg artery.

15. What is severe PAD or "critical limb ischemia"?

If PAD progresses to the point of severely reducing blood flow to the legs even at rest, then the survival of

PAD Pathophysiology

Claudication
Fatigue, discomfort, or pain that occurs in the leg muscles during exercise and that always resolves promptly with rest. This symptom usually occurs reproducibly at the same walking distance day-to-day, and can be considered as "angina of the legs." Claudication is a common symptom of PAD and results from blockages in the arteries that prevent blood, oxygen, and nutrients from reaching the working muscles.

Acute arterial occlusion (or acute limb ischemia [ALI])
A sudden and complete occlusion (blockage) of an artery in the leg. This presentation of PAD is quite uncommon and is typically due to either a blood clot (thrombus) traveling from a site upstream, such as from the heart, or the aortic or from a popliteal artery aneurysm to a more distant leg artery.

Gangrene

When tissue dies due to lack of blood flow. Gangrene is a sign of severe PAD, and if blood flow is not improved immediately, amputation may be required.

Critical limb ischemia (CLI)

One of the most severe manifestations of PAD in which the blood flow to the legs and feet is decreased to the point where there is pain, even at rest, wounds do not heal promptly, and tissue death (or "gangrene") occurs. Without prompt treatment, amputation may be necessary.

the leg itself may be threatened. Severe decreases in blood flow can cause pain in the foot or leg at rest (ischemic rest pain), a nonhealing skin wound, or **gangrene**. If blood flow is not improved immediately in such circumstances, then amputation may be required. Critical limb ischemia typically occurs when the blood pressure at the ankle is less than 50 mm Hg. This severe manifestation of PAD is termed **critical limb ischemia**, or simply CLI.

16. What causes gangrene of the foot?

Gangrene of the foot in the setting of PAD is due to such severely decreased blood flow that the skin, tissue, or bone dies. When blood flow is severely decreased and the protection of the skin is lost, infection can occur quickly and worsen within days. Gangrene of the foot occurs most commonly in patients whose PAD is left untreated for years, whose risk factors are poorly controlled, and whose PAD is not diagnosed in the earlier stages. Gangrene can occur with increased frequency in people with diabetes in whom the ability to feel skin injuries is lessened (a condition known as neuropathy) and in whom the ability to heal even minor foot trauma is impaired.

17. Does leg swelling indicate the presence of a blocked leg artery?

No, leg swelling is not a symptom of PAD alone. Leg swelling can be caused by many other medical problems, including thyroid disease, kidney disease, heart disease, and other diseases. The most common vascular reasons for leg swelling are poor blood flow in the leg veins (as occurs in people with "venous insufficiency" or who have suffered a prior deep vein thrombosis) or blocked lymph vessels, a condition called **lymphedema**.

Lymphedema

Leg swelling caused by blockages in the small lymphatic blood vessels.

18. Can a blocked vein cause PAD?

No, or almost never. Veins do not supply blood *to* the legs, although they do work to return blood from the legs to the heart. Very rarely, leg veins can be severely blocked due to a large amount of clot (a severe **deep vein thrombosis**, or DVT), and this blockage of blood *out* of the leg can impair the heart's ability to pump blood *into* the leg. This situation is called **phlegmasia cerulea dolens**, and when it occurs, the blood flow in the arteries to the leg may be so significantly reduced that it causes leg muscle pain even at rest. It is also worth noting that veins do not develop cholesterol plaque, unlike arteries.

19. Do varicose veins cause PAD?

No. Varicose veins are dilated veins. As veins dilate, they can be associated with discomfort if they are irritated (inflamed) or are under high pressure. Also, individuals with varicose veins can feel "heaviness" in their legs as the day passes or with prolonged standing. But, varicose veins do *not* cause PAD, and the discomfort of these veins is different than that of PAD.

20. Does infection cause PAD?

Although some studies have shown the presence of bacteria in cholesterol plaques in leg arteries, the data are unclear as to whether this is an insignificant association or a causative agent.

Deep vein thrombosis (DVT)
A blood clot in the deep veins of the leg. This disease is not related to PAD.

Phlegmasia cerulea dolens
A rare condition where DVT blockage of blood *out* of the leg impairs the heart's ability to pump blood *into* the leg. When this occurs, the blood flow to the leg arteries may cause muscle pain even at rest.

PAD Pathophysiology

PART THREE

Symptoms and Physical Findings of PAD

What is claudication?

What is a foot ulcer and can it be caused by PAD?

Can the arteries in my arms get blockages like those in leg arteries and cause pain?

More . . .

When you tell a physician or any health professional about how you feel, you are describing your symptoms. *When your physician or health professional examines your body, he or she is looking for evidence of health or disease from the* physical findings *of the examination. For individuals with PAD, the appearance of the legs and strength of the pulses may provide* physical findings *of artery blockage, whether symptoms are present or not.*

21. What are the symptoms of PAD?

The "classic" symptom of PAD is the "cramplike" leg muscle fatigue, discomfort, or pain that occurs in the buttock, thigh, or calf muscles with walking that reproducibly goes away 5–10 minutes after walking is stopped. The medical term for this discomfort is claudication. It is important to know that the majority of people with PAD do not have these classic symptoms. At least half of people with PAD have no recognizable leg symptoms of any kind.

A larger fraction of people with PAD (approximately 3–4 in 10) have atypical leg pain, which is described as leg symptoms that are not classic. This condition includes leg symptoms that occur both at rest or with exercise, or that do not resolve right away with rest. How can this be? As individuals age, there are *many* potential causes of leg discomfort, and these other causes may coexist with classic claudication. Some individuals have discomfort from arthritis or other orthopedic or podiatric conditions, neuropathy, gout, etc.

Mary's comment:

My symptoms were primarily muscle cramping, and I thought therefore that it was simply leg cramps. I tried to resolve my symptoms by exercising more to try and work the cramp out. However, it was apparent that this was not going to work and that the only relief I could get was when I stopped exercising and rested my leg. This was very frustrating because I truly wanted to believe it was a simple leg cramp and to continue exercising.

22. What is claudication?

Claudication, derived from the Latin word for "to limp," is the medical term for a specific discomfort in the leg muscles that occurs with exercise. Any leg muscle can be affected by claudication, but the buttocks, thighs, and calves are the most common locations of this discomfort. Some patients describe the discomfort as "pain," but most people experience claudication as a "heaviness," "cramping," "fatigue," or "numbness" within the leg muscles (**Figure 3**).

Note that claudication does *not* affect the joints, such as the hip, knee, or ankle. Claudication very rarely affects the foot or toes. Pain at these sites is much more likely to represent another disease.

One way to think of claudication accurately is to consider it similar to the discomfort that affects patients with coronary (heart) artery blockages. From this perspective, claudication is "angina of the legs."

23. Why do my muscles hurt when I exercise?

One or more blockages in the leg arteries may cause reduced blood flow to the working leg muscles. The response of the leg muscle to reduced oxygen is discomfort (claudication). This discomfort is similar to the

One way to think of claudication accurately is to consider it similar to the discomfort that affects patients with coronary (heart) artery blockages. From this perspective, claudication is "angina of the legs."

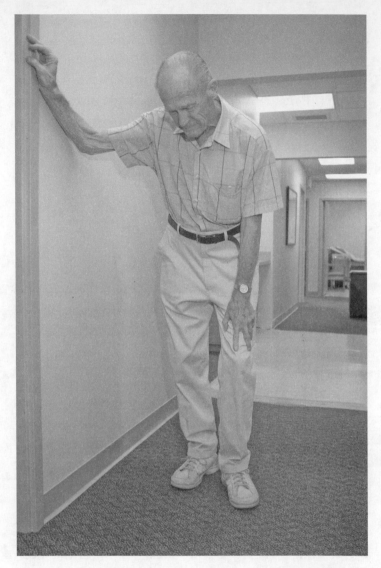

Figure 3 **Patient with claudication. (Courtesy of Medical Communications Media.)**

discomfort anyone would feel when the muscles are pushed beyond their capacity to work effectively. The difference is that people with PAD and claudication feel this discomfort at very low workloads associated with common activities every day.

24. Does darkening of the skin of the legs indicate PAD?

No, dark discoloration of the skin of a person's legs, especially near the lower calves or ankles, usually indicates a vein problem. Chronic (prolonged) swelling of the legs can lead to iron and protein leaking from the bloodstream into surrounding skin. The skin can become chronically inflamed from the stretching and the leakage of fluid that can occur for years. This inflammation can cause a dark color to develop, typically in the medial (inner) side of the leg above the ankle. If this finding is present, your doctor should evaluate you for **venous insufficiency** and may prescribe support hose or recommend a procedure to decrease the leakage of blood past abnormal vein valves. Such a problem can coexist in individuals with PAD, but it is an unrelated condition.

25. Are frequent cold feet or legs a sign of poor circulation from PAD?

Complaints of cold feet or legs are so common that this symptom cannot be considered specific for PAD. Individuals with PAD can experience cold lower extremities, especially when PAD is severe. But most people with cold legs do not have PAD.

26. What is a foot ulcer and can it be caused by PAD?

An **ulcer** is an area of tissue erosion that can occur on the skin of the foot in the setting of severe impairment of circulation from PAD (**Figure 4**). An ulcer due to PAD is painful and may be accompanied by infection, a situation that can be life threatening. Anyone with PAD who develops a foot ulcer should seek immediate

Venous insufficiency
A medical problem that occurs when leg veins are unable to function efficiently due to prior blockage or to the presence of leaky vein valves that impair the rapid return of blood to the heart.

Ulcer
The loss of a layer of skin tissue, due to injury, infection, damaged sensory nerves, or PAD. Skin ulcers, regardless of cause, are most dangerous in the presence of any severe impairment of blood flow, as occurs in some individuals with PAD.

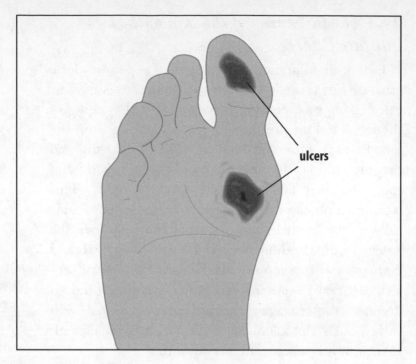

ulcers

Figure 4   Foot with ulcers.

medical attention and be considered for a procedure that improves blood flow to the foot. Other diseases such as diabetes can result in foot ulcers in people who have normal circulation; these ulcers are typically not painful but still require medical treatment.

27. Is hair loss or shiny skin on a person's legs a sign of PAD?

Older medical textbooks and some published "self-help" information still available to the public state that the loss of leg hair or presence of shiny skin on the legs is a sign of PAD. In general, this is a myth and there is not a strong relationship at all between either of these conditions and the presence of PAD. The loss of hair or shiny skin can also occur in people with normal leg circulation.

28. Can the arteries in my arms get blockages like those in leg arteries and cause pain?

Yes, cholesterol plaque can build up in your arm arteries and cause poor circulation and pain with exercise of the upper extremity. The pain typically involves a muscle of the arm and occurs after repeated movement; thus it is called arm claudication. The artery most commonly affected is the subclavian artery in the shoulder region.

29. Does PAD cause nocturnal leg cramps?

Nocturnal leg cramps are described as tension or tightness that occurs suddenly at night and may last up to 10 minutes. Although often associated with PAD, the exact cause of nocturnal leg cramps is unknown. There are conditions such as dehydration, inactivity, and electrolyte disturbances (such as abnormal levels of potassium or calcium) that may worsen this condition. Immediate relief of cramps is usually obtained by stretching the muscle. Regular exercise may reduce frequency of leg cramps. Quinine is no longer routinely prescribed for nocturnal leg cramps due to potential side effects.

30. Is restless leg syndrome caused by PAD?

Restless leg syndrome is a neurological condition that is characterized by the irresistible urge to move the leg. This condition should not be confused with nocturnal leg cramps, as restless leg syndrome is not accompanied by pain. There is no known link between restless leg syndrome and PAD.

PART FOUR

PAD
Diagnosis

What is an ankle-brachial index (ABI) test?

What is a duplex arterial ultrasound?

What is a catheter angiogram?

More . . .

If you are at risk of PAD based on your age, family history, or risk factors; if you have leg symptoms that make you suspicious that you might have PAD; or if you simply have decreased or absent ankle pulses, it is important that you seek care from a physician or other health professional to determine if you do have PAD. Establishing the PAD diagnosis is almost always easy, is nearly risk-free, and can be inexpensive.

31. How is PAD diagnosed?

All cardiovascular illnesses should be promptly diagnosed, and PAD is as important a diagnosis as any other heart or brain disease.

PAD is a very common cardiovascular illness. *All* cardiovascular illnesses should be promptly diagnosed, and PAD is as important a diagnosis as any other heart or brain disease. If present, PAD always defines an increased risk of heart attack and stroke, and it may define a risk of leg symptoms. Establishment of a prompt diagnosis can help avoid those rare instances in which amputation could become necessary. If you think you or a loved one may have PAD, seek prompt attention from a skilled doctor, physician's assistant, or nurse practitioner who can help determine if you do indeed have this illness. **Table 1** defines the groups of people who should definitely seek such attention.

Table 1   Individuals at Risk for Lower Extremity Peripheral Artery Disease

• Age less than 50 years with diabetes and on other atherosclerosis risk factor (smoking, dyslipidemia, hypertension, or hyperhomocysteinemia)
• Age 50 to 69 years and a history of smoking or diabetes
• Age 70 years and older
• Leg symptoms with exertion (suggestive of claudication) or ischemic rest pain Abnormal lower extremity pulse examination
• Known atherosclerotic coronary, carotid, or renal artery disease

The clinician will evaluate your medical history, including your risk factors for PAD (a history of tobacco use, diabetes, high blood cholesterol, high blood pressure, or a family history of coronary heart disease or PAD). The clinician will also ask you questions to determine if you have leg symptoms suggestive of PAD (such as exertional leg muscle pain, nonhealing wounds, or gangrene). Your heart and pulses (from your neck to your toes) will be evaluated. Then you will likely undergo a simple blood pressure test at the ankles, called an **ankle-brachial index**, or ABI, **test** (see Question 32). These simple tests are all that is required for more than 90% of individuals with PAD. Sometimes, as described in the following questions, more advanced ultrasound or imaging tests may be ordered (especially in people with more severe leg symptoms).

In other words, establishing a PAD diagnosis is risk-free, easy, and need not be expensive. All healthcare providers should be equipped to help you answer the question, "Do I have PAD?"

32. What is an ankle-brachial index (ABI) test?

Since PAD is defined by the presence of blockages in the arteries that supply the legs, it is not surprising that the most common diagnostic test for PAD measures the blood pressure at the legs (below an artery blockage) and compares this pressure to the blood pressure at the arms. In healthy individuals, the higher blood pressure measurement, the systolic pressure (for example, the "120" in a blood pressure of 120/80 mm Hg), is always slightly higher at the ankles compared to either arm.

The ankle-brachial index, or simply ABI, test is performed by a doctor, nurse, or trained ultrasound

Ankle-brachial index (ABI) test

A noninvasive, safe, and inexpensive blood pressure test that compares the higher (systolic) blood pressures that are recorded at the arms and ankles. This test is usually required for all individuals with PAD.

PAD Diagnosis

Toe-brachial index

A test that is used to diagnose PAD that is performed by measuring the relative blood pressures in the great toes and arms. This test is especially useful in individuals with diabetes and those in whom the ABI test is not accurate.

Duplex arterial ultrasound

A noninvasive test that uses sound waves (ultrasound) to measure how blood moves through arteries and that can define the presence of artery blockages without exposure to X-rays.

Computerized tomographic (CT) angiogram

A noninvasive method of looking at arteries inside the body using a donut shaped X-ray camera and intravenous dye. Two- and three-dimensional, highly detailed images of arteries are possible with this method.

technician (sonographer) who places a standard blood pressure cuff on both upper arms and also on both legs just above the ankles. The systolic blood pressure is then recorded at each of the four sites. The blood pressure is recorded from *two* arteries at each ankle. The higher arm blood pressure is always considered to be the most accurate because artery blockages can less frequently be present in an arm artery of someone with PAD. Then, the four ankle blood pressures are used in calculating the ABI.

The ratio of the ankle to arm blood pressure is always greater than 1.10 in healthy individuals.

Although there is more than one method of determining which of the four ratios is used in determining a person's ABI, any ABI value less than 0.90 is considered abnormal and indicates PAD. Values between 0.90 and 1.10 are considered borderline and are non-diagnostic according to current standards (though even these minimally decreased values may demonstrate some future risk). Depending on whether leg symptoms are present, the clinician may repeat the ABI test on another occasion or request an alternative test, such as measurement of the great toe pressure (**toe-brachial index**), or the clinician may perform a leg **duplex arterial ultrasound**, leg **computerized tomographic (CT) angiogram**, or **magnetic resonance (MR) angiogram**.

The ABI test is useful in nearly all people, but there are limitations to every medical diagnostic test, and this is true for the ABI test as well (**Figure 5**). For a small group of individuals with PAD, the arteries at the ankle may be insufficiently compressible by the blood pressure cuff due to advanced age, longstanding diabetes, treatment with immunosuppressive medications for organ transplants, and other reasons. In these individuals, the ABI value may be in excess of 1.30, and such values are not normal. For these individuals, an alternative PAD test should be considered (such as a toe-brachial index test or a duplex arterial ultrasound test, as discussed in Question 34).

Magnetic resonance (MR) angiogram

A noninvasive method of looking at arteries inside the body using MR imaging. The body is passed into a long tube and an intravenous medication is injected to permit the arteries to be visible.

PAD Diagnosis

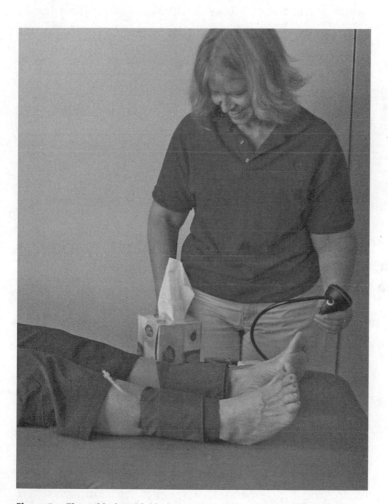

Figure 5   The ankle-brachial index (ABI) test. (Courtesy of PAD Coalition.)

33. What is an exercise ABI stress test?

It was once common for vascular specialists to evaluate individuals with PAD in the absence of measurements provided by an exercise stress test "because patients with PAD can't walk." Yet, since the main function of the legs is, in fact, to walk and because we all feel discomfort differently, it can be extremely challenging for individuals (or their spouses or family members) or their physicians to accurately know the degree of impairment that exists by a casual office discussion alone. Some patients may complain little to their families or physicians but may in fact be severely impaired. Other patients may complain a lot but may in fact have tremendous reserve and not need to undergo a risky procedure that once seemed necessary. And other patients may have PAD that—on first review—would seem to be the major impediment to walking, but testing may show that another medical problem (such as knee or hip arthritis, or shortness of breath) is in fact much more important.

Knowledge of how far an individual can walk can provide a benchmark of today's leg health and can markedly change patient and physician perceptions of "walking ability." A treadmill stress test can serve as the first step toward achieving a therapeutic "exercise prescription" within a PAD rehabilitation program. Heart stress tests also may provide key information about associated risk of **coronary heart disease**, which is a key issue for all individuals with PAD.

Treadmill tests for patients with PAD and claudication use much less intense progressive workloads than are used for patients evaluated for heart disease. They record the time of onset of specific leg symptoms, the presence of associated heart (anginal) symptoms, and

Coronary heart disease

Heart disease caused when the arteries that supply the heart are narrowed by plaque buildup, which can lead to both angina and heart attack.

the total walking time. Continuous ECG (electrocardiogram) monitoring is a very useful, but optional, component of these tests. When a treadmill is not available, this test can also be done by asking the patient to perform 10 or more toe raises. For either form of the exercise ABI test, the patient undergoes a recording of the ABI at rest and after exercise (**Figure 6**). In normal individuals, the arm and ankle blood pressures rise together and maintain a nearly equal relationship with exertion. In contrast, in patients with PAD, exercise

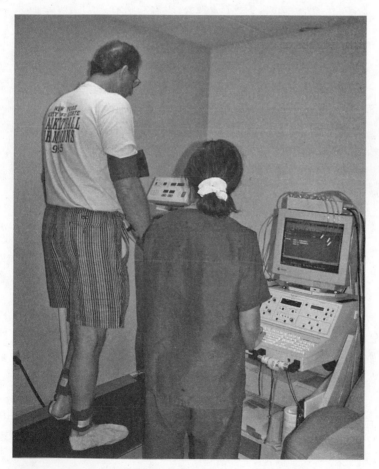

Figure 6   The exercise ankle-brachial index stress test. (Courtesy of American College of Cardiology.)

31

produces a diagnostic fall in the ABI in the affected leg immediately after exercise.

Also, the exercise ABI test can be helpful in distinguishing a walking impairment that can occur in individuals with lumbar spinal disease (known as pseudoclaudication) from the discomfort that is caused by PAD.

Mary's comment:

I was a little uncomfortable when I found out I needed to have a "stress test." I had taken cardio stress tests in the past and did not make it through them because of leg aching. At that time, however, the practitioners did not make the association between my reason for quitting the test and the possibility of claudication because I had gone a greater distance than one would have seen when questioning a diagnosis of PAD. The ABI stress test was very easy to take and the practitioner was very reassuring that I would not be pushed past the point of an onset of pain.

34. What is a duplex arterial ultrasound?

All individuals with PAD deserve an accurate diagnosis associated with a measurement that defines the severity of their disease.

All individuals with PAD deserve an accurate diagnosis associated with a measurement that defines the severity of their disease. While this can usually be provided by an ABI test alone, the ABI test does not provide information regarding the exact site of any leg artery blockage. Not all individuals with PAD need to know the details of their leg anatomy and the site of such blockages. For example, individuals with no leg symptoms or mild symptoms (over half of those with PAD) gain no benefit from any additional diagnostic testing beyond the ABI test.

However, individuals with significant leg symptoms can benefit from knowing the site(s) and severity of any artery blockage. This information can guide the patient and physician together to different treatment choices. For example, an individual with complex PAD blockages in more than one location may most benefit from an exercise program, whereas an individual with one severe narrowing in a high (iliac or femoral) artery near the groin may benefit from an angioplasty.

Duplex arterial ultrasound uses sound waves to map the site of an artery blockage (**Figure 7**). A handheld probe is placed on the skin, and sound waves can define the size of the artery and its branches, and they can measure the velocity of blood flow. When artery blood flow markedly increases, it is commonly a sign of a severe blockage. This test can map most of the arteries from the groin to the toes and is often used to map the diameter and blood flow in the aorta. Ultrasound is useful in detecting aneurysms (a ballooning of the walls) of the aorta and of the iliac, femoral, or popliteal arteries. Some individuals may be so large that ultrasound cannot adequately penetrate the abdominal fat to provide an adequate picture. For these individuals, an MRA (see Question 36) or CTA (see Question 38) may be needed to provide this more detailed information.

There is no known risk to using ultrasound to map artery size or to measure blood flow.

35. What is transcutaneous oximetry?

One major challenge for some patients with severe PAD is to determine if a foot or ankle skin wound has adequate blood flow to heal. There are few medical challenges more debilitating and frustrating than the pain, topical care, and impaired freedom to walk associated with many months of care for a nonhealing wound.

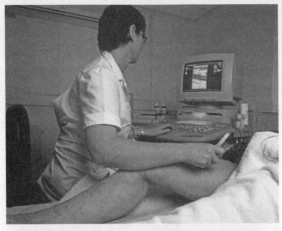

(a)

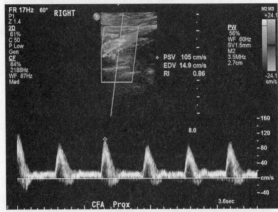

(b)

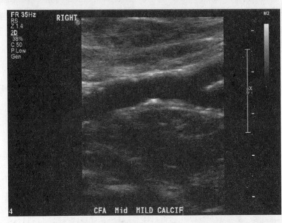

(c)

Figure 7 (a) A duplex arterial ultrasound test. (© James King-Holmes/Photo Researchers, Inc.) (b) This panel shows the dividing of the common femoral artery, with no blockages in view. (c) This panel shows the measurements of blood velocity that confirm that no blockage is present. (See color plates A and B.)

For this situation, mere measurement of the site of a blockage does not truly grade how much net blood flow is provided to the skin near such wounds. Some individuals may also have normal leg arteries but impaired blood flow to the skin or toes because of a blood clot or cholesterol crystals that float downstream from the heart or aorta to the skin or toes. Thus, the physician may need to directly measure the blood flow to the skin.

This measurement is particularly important for the assessment of patients with critical limb ischemia (CLI) who have pain at rest, skin ulcerations, and/or impending gangrene. The net delivery of oxygen to the skin tissue is measured by the **transcutaneous oximetry (TcPO$_2$) test,** which uses oxygen-sensing electrodes. These electrodes are attached to the skin of the chest, which almost always has normal blood supply, and at calf or foot sites to directly measure the local skin oxygen delivery. TcPO$_2$ measurements inform the patient and physician of the realistic potential for wound healing at the affected sites. Normal TcPO$_2$ values are usually greater than 50–60 mm Hg; in contrast, TcPO$_2$ values less than 20–30 mm Hg suggest severe local ischemia and bode poorly for future wound healing. There is no risk associated with performance of this test.

Transcutaneous oximetry (TcPO$_2$) test

A test that uses oxygen-sensing electrodes to measure the delivery of oxygen to the skin tissue. This test is used often in individuals with slow-healing skin wounds.

36. What is an MRA?

Wouldn't it be great if one could obtain detailed pictures of the leg arteries without any (or with minimal) risk? Fortunately, this is possible with magnetic resonance (MR) angiography (**Figure 8**). Most MR angiograms (or MRAs) are performed using contrast-enhancement in which a substance called gadolinium is injected just before the scan is taken. Gadolinium permits the moving

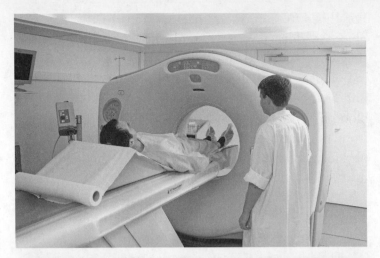

(a)

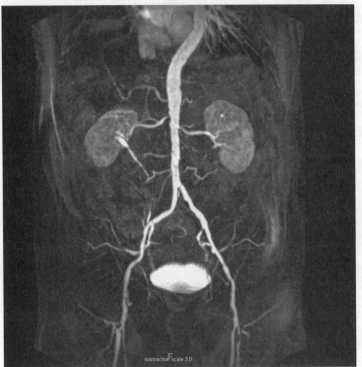

(b)

Figure 8 (a) A magnetic resonance (MR) angiogram test. (© AJ Photos/Photo Researchers, Inc.) (b) This is an angiogram that shows the aorta, two kidneys with their artery supplies, and the bifurcation of the aorta into both common iliac arteries. (See color plate C.)

blood to be seen in greater detail. MRA is a useful technique for assessing the aorta, renal arteries, and leg arteries, as well as the arteries to the brain.

The MR camera is a long tube into which the person being examined is placed. It is both noisy and physically confining. Most MR scans require approximately 40–60 minutes of scanning time. Thus, some individuals may feel claustrophobic inside the scanner. For these individuals, use of a sedative can be helpful. Individuals with implanted metallic devices, such as pacemakers and defibrillators, cannot safely have pictures taken in these scanning machines.

37. Are there side effects to MRA?

While there are no known side effects of the magnetism that is used to take MRA pictures, there are safety concerns that can affect individuals who undergo MR scans. Most notably, people with abnormal kidney function should usually not undergo MRA if gadolinium is to be used as a contrast agent, as this carries a risk of development of a rare but serious and irreversible disease called nephrogenic systemic sclerosis. The mechanism by which gadolinium might cause this reaction remains unknown, but the disease is associated with fibrosis (scarring) of the skin and body organs. If this reaction occurs, there is no known treatment.

38. What is a CTA?

Another method of looking inside the body to evaluate the blood vessels uses a computerized tomographic (CT) scanner that takes cross-sectional slices of the body. These slices can then be reconstructed to form a three-dimensional internal view of the inner body structures. When the arteries are imaged in this way, the pictures are called a CT angiogram, or simply a CTA (**Figure 9**). Current CT scanners produce highly detailed three-dimensional angiographic images of the aorta, brain, renal arteries, and lower extremity arteries. The CTA technique requires the administration of 100–150 cc of iodinated contrast and thus carries some risk for patients with renal insufficiency. The CTA technique also uses radiation, and the exposure to any radiation carries some finite adverse risk. The CTA technique maintains one advantage over the MRA technique, as metal stents may be imaged with CTA and in-stent **restenosis** detected.

39. What is a catheter angiogram?

A **catheter angiogram** is an invasive test that uses special catheters (tubes) that are passed through the skin, usually from the groin, into the arteries (**Figure 10**). Injection of a **radiopaque dye** permits X-rays to provide a very detailed picture of the size and direction of each artery. An angiogram usually takes approximately one hour.

40. Are there side effects from an angiogram?

Yes. While an angiogram can be extremely useful and is very safe, adverse effects can occur. These include damage to the artery that is used to gain access to the circulation, bleeding, pain at the site of the angiogram skin puncture, an allergy to the contrast dye, or kidney failure from the dye.

41. What is an angioplasty?

An angioplasty is a procedure used to treat artery blockages. An angioplasty is usually performed just after an angiogram. The treating physician will thread a small tube (catheter) that has an inflatable balloon at its tip

Restenosis

A recurring narrowing of an artery after any corrective treatment such as angioplasty or bypass surgery.

Catheter angiogram

An invasive test that uses special tubes (catheters) that are passed through the skin, usually from the groin, into the arteries. A solution that is opaque on X-Rays (a "dye") is then injected through the tube into the arteries so they appear clearly on an X-ray. An angiogram usually takes approximately 1 hour.

Radiopaque dye

The dye injected into arteries during an angiogram to permit X-rays to provide a detailed picture of their size and direction.

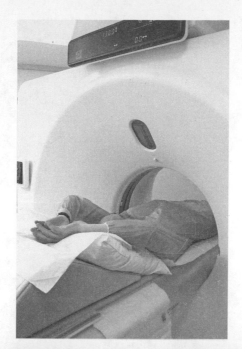

(a)

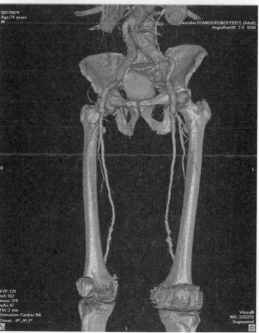

(b)

Figure 9 **(a)** A computerized tomographic (CT) angiogram test. (© Laurent/Claudine/Photo Researchers, Inc.) **(b)** A CT test result that shows stents in the common iliac arteries and superficial femoral arteries in each leg that travel in the thigh and behind each knee. (See color plates D and E.)

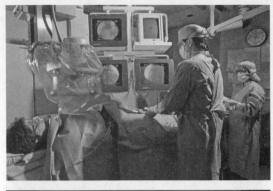

(a)

(b)

Figure 10 (a) A catheter-based angiogram. (© Gary Hansen/ Phototake/Alamy Images) (b) Test results. (Courtesy of Christopher P. Molgaard, MD, Lahey Clinic Medical Center) (See color plate F.)

This technique is so helpful that most patients can avoid a surgical procedure and have an artery opened at much lower risk.

(**Figure 11**). This catheter is passed into the artery, and the balloon is inflated (blown up) to widen a narrowed or completely blocked artery. This technique is so helpful that most patients can avoid a surgical procedure and have an artery opened at much lower risk.

Angioplasty opens an artery, but the living tissue of the artery can constrict or rapidly renarrow after it is first treated. This occurrence is called restenosis. Physicians

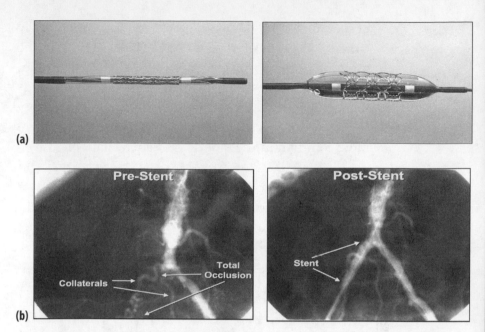

Figure 11 (a) An angioplasty balloon catheter and stent. (b) Angiogram of bilaterial artery stent results (before and after stent placement).

can sometimes place a tiny metallic coil, called a stent, to serve as a rigid framework to keep the artery open. Once implanted, such a stent is permanent and is not later removed.

Angioplasty, with or without stent placement, does not "fix" a blood vessel, and, although often very helpful, this procedure does not reverse PAD nor prolong life. Angioplasty of leg arteries can be used to treat claudication or to improve blood flow for individuals with critical limb ischemia (CLI; pain at rest due to very severe artery blockages, nonhealing skin wounds, or gangrene). It can help patients with CLI to avoid amputation.

Angioplasty is not a permanent treatment. The ability of a physician to open an artery depends on the length

41

of the blockage (shorter blockages are more easily treated), the site of the blockage (blockages near the groin or in the aorta, iliac arteries, or femoral arteries are more easily treated compared with those in the mid-thigh and below the knee), and the stiffness of the artery (as when due to calcification, and tough blockages are more common in the elderly or diabetic patients).

If your physician proposes to use angioplasty, with or without a stent, to treat your PAD, you will want to ask:

"What is the likelihood of success in opening the artery in my case?"

"What is the expected likelihood that the artery will stay open in 6 months, 12 months, or in 2 to 5 years?"

"Are there other treatments that I might consider instead of, or in addition to, angioplasty?

Mary's comment:

Although my artery was approximately 93% occluded, I was fortunate because there appeared to be only one blockage and the site was good for this procedure. I had an angioplasty with stent placement in my left iliac artery. As soon as I was allowed to get up and walk, I was amazed to find that I had absolutely no pain at all with walking or resting.

PART FIVE

PAD Risk Factors

Does cigarette smoking cause PAD?

Does high blood pressure cause PAD?

Is diabetes a risk factor for PAD?

More . . .

Your arteries are literally the "rivers of life" that nourish your brain, heart, major body organs, arms, and legs. The arteries provide the tissues with the ability to live and to heal.

Arteries do not fail randomly. They have an extraordinary ability to perform their function through 5, 6, 7, or 8 decades of human life. Arteries become damaged when they are exposed to factors that humans did not face during the millennium of our evolution: tobacco smoke; persistent high blood sugar, as occurs with diabetes; marked elevations in blood cholesterol; or the mechanical stress of high blood pressure. Further, once plaque forms, rupture of the surface of the plaque can cause a clot to form and suddenly block all flow, causing heart attack and stroke.

You are offered the gift of but one body, with its arteries, during your lifetime. You can choose to ignore the impact of these modifiable risk factors or you can choose to provide your arteries with protection from ongoing damage. If you protect your arteries, they will protect you. You will survive, and you will do so with greater joy and less suffering.

42. Are there factors that predispose a person to development of PAD?

Yes, as mentioned in Question 5, the risk factors for PAD include smoking, diabetes, high blood pressure, and high cholesterol (**Table 2**). When you were born, your arteries were open and the lining was smooth. This lining is fragile and anything that damages it (the risk factors) can make you much more vulnerable to suffering from PAD.

Table 2   Risk of Developing Lower Extremity PAD

Risk Factors	Relative Risk
Smoking	2–4
Diabetes	2–4
Hypertension	1.5–2.5
Hypercholesterolemia	1–2
Hyperhomocysteinemia	2–3
C-Reactive Protein	2–2.25

43. Does cigarette smoking cause PAD?

Yes, smoking is one of the most potent risk factors for developing PAD. The many chemicals inhaled with smoke (or absorbed into the body when tobacco is chewed) cause arteries to be directly damaged and cholesterol to build up in the artery wall. Smoking causes the blood vessels to constrict and causes the blood to become much more likely to clot. Individuals who smoke, even a little, face a much higher likelihood of their leg pain worsening or having their PAD worsen so much that amputation may be required. Smoking makes PAD more severe so that the chance of needing leg artery bypass surgery increases.

Smoking causes the blood vessels to constrict and causes the blood to become much more likely to clot.

A woman who smokes faces a risk of PAD equal to that of a man 10 years older.

44. Is diabetes a risk factor for PAD?

Yes, diabetes is one of the most potent risk factors for PAD. It is estimated that almost half of patients with diabetes will develop cholesterol plaque in the leg arteries. It is important for all patients with diabetes to keep their blood sugar under control in order to prevent eye and kidney problems.

45. Does having prediabetes predispose to PAD?

Yes, the prediabetic state, frequently due to a group of factors called the **metabolic syndrome**, increases the risk of development of PAD. This metabolic syndrome typically involves an elevated blood sugar near the diabetic range, low good cholesterol, high fat (triglycerides), and high blood pressure. The underlying problem is an inability of insulin (the hormone secreted from the pancreas that controls blood sugar) to work properly.

46. Does high blood pressure cause PAD?

Yes, high blood pressure (hypertension) increases the risk of developing PAD. It is thought that the high pressure in the arteries causes dysfunction of the artery wall, resulting in development of cholesterol plaque. Even a very small increase in blood pressure from the normal range can greatly worsen your risk of heart attack and stroke, as well as PAD.

47. Does high cholesterol cause PAD?

Yes, a high blood cholesterol level increases the risk for development of cholesterol plaques in the leg arteries. Patients with extremely high bad cholesterol (low-density lipoprotein) levels are at much higher risk than those with lower levels.

48. Does homocysteine cause PAD?

Homocysteine is a natural amino acid, or building block of proteins, in your body. Like cholesterol, there is a normal amount of homocysteine that is needed to

---

Metabolic syndrome

A high-risk condition in which a group of multiple risk factors coexist. These risk factors include an elevated blood sugar near the diabetic range, low good cholesterol (HDL), high triglyceride levels, and high blood pressure. The underlying problem is an inability of insulin (the hormone secreted from the pancreas that controls blood sugar) to work properly. Metabolic syndrome increases the risk of development of PAD.

Patients with extremely high bad cholesterol (low-density lipoprotein) levels are at much higher risk than those with lower levels.

maintain good health. However, homocysteine at high levels in the blood can directly damage the artery wall or cause blood clots. Elevation of homocysteine is a weak risk factor for development of PAD. For many years, due to early studies that suggested that lowering homocysteine might be useful, blood tests for this substance were commonly performed and certain B vitamins were prescribed to lower homocysteine levels. More recent and better scientific studies have now confirmed that use of these vitamins to lower blood levels of homocysteine is not useful in preventing heart attack and stroke.

Homocysteine

A natural amino acid in the body that is needed to maintain good health. Too high levels in the blood, however, can damage artery walls or cause blood clots, and may be a risk factor for developing PAD. There is no evidence that treating elevated homocysteine levels has any beneficial therapeutic effect.

49. What is C-reactive protein?

C-reactive protein, also known as high-sensitivity C-reactive protein (or hs-CRP), is a protein that travels in the bloodstream and is increased when there is any illness that causes inflammation. For example, C-reactive protein is commonly elevated in people who have an infection such as the common cold. Research studies have shown an association between increased levels of C-reactive protein and both heart attack and stroke.

50. Is C-reactive protein associated with PAD?

Yes, C-reactive protein is associated with PAD. However, many people without PAD have elevated levels of C-reactive protein, and many individuals with PAD have normal levels of C-reactive protein. Thus, this blood test is not very specific for PAD and is usually not used in the diagnosis of PAD or in the assessment of PAD severity.

While scientists continue to investigate how C-reactive protein is made in the body and what its functions are, there is no substantial information to suggest that C-reactive protein causes PAD.

PAD Risk Factors

51. Is there a gene that causes PAD?

At present, there is no single gene or set of genes identified in humans that is associated with PAD. There are, however, genes associated with atherosclerosis in the heart arteries, and since heart arteries are related to atherosclerosis in leg arteries, it is likely that genes will be identified that will predict personal risk of PAD.

PART SIX

Heart Attack, Stroke, and Limb Loss in Individuals with PAD

Am I at risk of heart attack if I have PAD?

Am I at risk of stroke if I have PAD?

Am I at risk of losing my leg if I have PAD?

More . . .

A core value that is central to all "best clinical care" is the honest sharing between patients and physicians of the realistic risks faced by the patient and family. Current information has clarified that, regardless of how common PAD is in so many communities, few members of the public (who have PAD or who are at risk of PAD) are aware of the tangible high risk of heart attack, stroke, amputation, and death that is present for all affected individuals. In the United States and Canada, a public survey conducted in 2006 demonstrated that less than one in four adults who were at risk of PAD due to age, risk factors, and leg symptoms had any awareness that PAD existed as a common disease. Of the one in four who were aware of PAD, even fewer were knowledgeable that PAD causes disability (claudication), heart attack, stroke, or amputation.

This risk is so important that most national and international PAD treatment guidelines mandate that treatments to lower this risk be considered the very first and top priority for any affected patient.

52. Am I at risk of heart attack if I have PAD?

Yes. Individuals with PAD, when caused by atherosclerosis, face as high—or higher—a risk of heart attack as an individual with known heart artery blockages who has survived a first heart attack. This risk is increased five- to seven-fold compared to someone without PAD. Because the same risk factors that cause blockages in leg arteries are likely to create plaque (blockages) in heart arteries, it is wise to assume that the risk is high and to start treatments to lower risk right away. These treatments should be maintained for a lifetime.

Mary's comment:

Since my risk for heart attack is increased because of my PAD diagnosis, I am more determined to follow my medication regimen as well as to watch my diet and increase my exercise. I know that there is no cure for PAD, but I am intent on doing what I can to prevent the blockage from increasing.

53. Am I at risk of heart attack after leg artery surgery if I have PAD?

Yes. While different vascular surgical procedures carry differing risks, all open surgical operations usually carry a 2–4% risk of heart attack within the first 30 days of the procedure. This risk is due to the stress associated with the surgical procedure and cannot currently be entirely abolished. The risk can be measured in some individuals by performance of a **heart stress test** before the leg surgical procedure. Often, such a stress test will use medications to speed the heart or to change heart artery blood flow instead of using a treadmill walking protocol. For patients who plan to undergo elective leg artery operations, a very positive (abnormal) heart stress test may lead your physician to recommend use of additional heart protective medications or for you to undergo a heart angiogram. All individuals with PAD should ask their doctor if they should continue to take **aspirin** or clopidogrel (Plavix) and if they should consider using **beta blockers** and/or **statin** medication.

The risk of heart attack and/or stroke does not resolve when your leg artery surgery is done. This risk continues throughout your life.

Heart Attack, Stroke, and Limb Loss in Individuals with PAD

Heart stress test

A test designed to measure if there are severe heart (coronary) artery blockages. Such a stress test can be performed using either treadmill or bicycle exercise, or by using medications that increase heart rate and heart function instead of exercise for individuals with PAD who may not be able to walk or run vigorously.

Aspirin

Acetylsalicylic acid, or ASA, is a non-prescription, anti-inflammatory medication that is used to reduce pain and fever. But, this medication is also proven to prevent blood from clotting in the arteries, and thus lowers the risk of heart attack or stroke in individuals who are at risk.

Beta blockers (β-blockers)

A class of antihypertensive medications that lower blood pressure and lower the risk of heart attack.

Statin

A class of cholesterol-lowering drugs that is best proven to lower rates of heart attack, stroke, or death.

All national and international recommendations for care of people with PAD state that patients should be offered a maximal program of risk reduction therapies without a need for additional stress testing.

54. Should I have a cardiac (heart) stress test?

For most individuals with PAD, the mere establishment of a PAD diagnosis will place you in a high-risk group for heart attack and stroke, and performance of a stress test does not change that risk. This is because even small artery blockages carry the same risk of heart attack as the most serious ones. Stress tests only identify the most severe artery blockages. Thus, all national and international recommendations for care of people with PAD state that patients should be offered a maximal program of risk reduction therapies without a need for additional stress testing.

Even if the stress test were positive (especially in people without any heart symptoms), there is almost never any procedure needed that will further improve your health beyond treating your risk factors. Thus, for most people with PAD who do *not* have heart symptoms (such as chest pain [angina] or shortness of breath with exercise), there is no need for a stress test to be performed.

On the other hand, if you do have PAD and some symptoms that might be due to coronary heart disease (such as chest pain or shortness of breath when exercising), you may benefit from a test that can determine more precisely if these symptoms deserve specific treatment.

If your physician plans to prescribe a supervised exercise program to improve your claudication, then he/she will likely ask you to exercise on a treadmill while monitoring you for heart symptoms, observing your ECG (electrical heart tracing), and measuring your ankle blood pressures before and after exercise. This information can help the doctor create a safe exercise program for you.

If it is recommended that you undergo an operative vascular surgical procedure, you will likely be asked to undergo a cardiac stress test, using either a treadmill or medications, to test your heart's ability to stay healthy during and after the operation.

55. What are the types of stress tests?

There are many forms of stress tests, and your physician is best positioned to determine if you need such a test and to determine which type would best answer the questions that can guide your future health.

For individuals with mild PAD (no leg symptoms or minimal claudication), a treadmill stress test can safely be used to determine your exercise capacity.

For individuals who have trouble walking due to either claudication or critical limb ischemia, a pharmacologic stress test or chemical stress test can be performed. In these tests, a medication (such as adenosine or dobutamine) can be used either to dilate the heart arteries or to speed the heart's contractions in order to mimic exercise. Then, either an echocardiogram (an ultrasound picture of the heart) or a nuclear scan can be used to view the heart muscle function and heart blood flow to determine if heart artery blockages are present.

56. Am I at risk of stroke if I have PAD?

Yes. Individuals with PAD, when caused by atherosclerosis, face as high a risk of stroke as individuals with known blockages in the carotid arteries or individuals who have survived a stroke. Because the same risk factors that cause blockages in the leg arteries are likely to create plaque (blockages) in carotid or brain arteries, it is wise to assume that the risk is high and to start treatments to lower risk right away. These treatments should be maintained for a lifetime.

57. Am I at risk of losing my leg if I have PAD?

Yes. But for nearly all individuals with PAD, this risk is extremely low. Less than 5% of people with PAD will ever face a real risk of losing a foot or leg. This risk is increased in people who smoke, have diabetes, or have restricted access to health care. The risk that is created by smoking, in particular, cannot be overemphasized. Smoking causes the arteries of the leg to both narrow and clot, and smoking adversely affects both angioplasty and bypass treatments so that they are much more likely to fail.

For individuals with severe PAD and critical limb ischemia, it is extremely important for foot care to be provided daily, for the feet to be routinely inspected, for any wounds to be reported to the doctor, for infection to be treated promptly, and for smoking to be stopped completely. Amputation can be prevented or delayed by taking these measures.

Finally, once an individual has been successfully treated for critical limb ischemia, it is important to maintain doctor visits, foot inspections, and proper foot care for the rest of his or her life. The risk of losing a foot can be markedly diminished, but it can never be fully abolished.

Smoking causes the arteries of the leg to both narrow and clot, and smoking adversely affects both angioplasty and bypass treatments so that they are much more likely to fail.

PART SEVEN

Lowering Risk: Treatment of Atherosclerosis Risk Factors and Use of Antithrombotic (Anticlotting) Medications

Should I lower my cholesterol if I have PAD?

How can I quit smoking? When should I begin my efforts to quit smoking?

Can I prevent a heart attack or stroke by using aspirin or other antithrombotic (anticlotting) medications?

More . . .

Individuals with PAD of any severity are at increased risk for heart attack, stroke, and amputation, but this risk can be managed effectively. It is possible to take many actions, most easy, that can provide some reassurance of safety. You have the opportunity, in partnership with your doctor and family, to protect your body, which both offers you shelter and transportation for the days of your life. If the task seems challenging, it is appropriate to ask for help from family, friends, and clinicians so that any perceived burden is lightened.

Lower your risk. Live your life. Do so with peace of mind.

58. Is there a cure for PAD?

Unfortunately there is at present no cure for PAD. The following questions discuss methods to prevent progression of disease in the legs and to improve lifestyle as well as methods to reduce the risk of heart attack, stroke, and amputation associated with PAD.

59. Should I lower my cholesterol if I have PAD?

Yes, and you should ideally do so immediately. Cholesterol levels can be lowered via combinations of diet, exercise, and medications. The method you choose to achieve this goal should be discussed with your physician. Action should begin the moment a PAD diagnosis is offered. Success will be achieved and will be sustained for life.

The national and international PAD medical care guidelines document why the most effective approach to lowering cholesterol levels is to use a statin medication (also called an HMG-CoA reductase inhibitor). While diet and exercise should also be components of any plan to sustain good health, these behavioral interventions take time and diligence, and even then, they may not lower cholesterol to levels associated with the greatest safety.

Patients with PAD who have never had a heart attack and/or stroke are considered to be at the same risk for a future heart and/or stroke as those who have already had this cardiovascular problem. In decades past, physicians and the public tended to measure the total blood cholesterol, and treatments were designed to lower this total cholesterol level. In contrast, modern information has shown that it is *not* the total cholesterol value that best predicts progressive PAD or heart attack. Instead, the best predictor of heart attack and stroke in individuals with PAD, as for individuals with coronary heart disease, is the low-density lipoprotein (LDL) cholesterol. The LDL cholesterol is often called the "bad cholesterol," as this is the fraction of cholesterol that directly blocks heart arteries.

Aggressive reduction of LDL cholesterol with a target goal of less than 100 mg/dL is recommended for all patients with PAD, no matter how severe (including those with no recognized symptoms). A lower LDL cholesterol value of less than 70 mg/dL is optimal and is recommended for those individuals with PAD who are at very high risk. Individuals at very high risk include patients with an uncontrolled risk factor, such as ongoing smoking, poorly controlled diabetes, or blood pressure that is not at target goals. Other individuals at very high risk can be defined by a medical history of atherosclerotic disease in locations other than the legs, such as in the heart or brain arteries. Because lowering cholesterol with medication is both safe and effective for most people, and because there is

Many physicians believe that every patient with PAD should strive for an LDL cholesterol level of less than 70 mg/dL.

no evidence that achieving lower cholesterol has any harm, many physicians believe that every patient with PAD should strive for an LDL cholesterol level of less than 70 mg/dL.

Mary's comment:

Since my diagnosis and stent placement, I have been able to keep my cholesterol low by following a total plan recommended by my physician. My total cholesterol level is significantly lower, my LDL is lower, and my HDL has increased.

60. Should I use statin medications to lower my cholesterol if I have PAD?

Yes, for nearly all individuals with PAD, regardless of their starting cholesterol measurement, statin medications have been shown to improve rates of heart attack, stroke, and death. While all high-quality cholesterol treatments should include an emphasis on diet, weight loss, and nonmedication approaches to normalizing blood cholesterol, most individuals benefit from statin drugs as well.

Individuals who use statin medications should also make realistic attempts to lose weight, to exercise, and to modify their diet to one that is "heart healthy."

61. Don't statin drugs cause muscle pain? I already have leg pain! What should I do?

Statin medications are among the safest medications available to treat a series of dangerous diseases that are known to cause heart attack, stroke, amputation, and death, and to markedly worsen quality of life. Yet, as for any medication, a small fraction of individuals may suffer an occasional adverse effect. For statin medications, it has long been known that a small fraction of individuals might feel muscle discomfort during treatment, even in the absence of PAD. This discomfort is rarely dangerous.

How can a patient with PAD determine if a statin medication is causing leg discomfort? Well, this is not easy. First, almost all adults feel leg muscle fatigue or pain from time to time. Since leg muscle pain, PAD, and statin use are all now quite common, it is challenging to know with certainty if a statin is indeed the cause of muscle pain. There is a real price paid if this statin–muscle pain relationship is assumed to be true and the medication is discontinued, thus depriving the patient of potential benefits.

If you experience the onset of a new type of leg or diffuse muscle pain upon beginning statin therapy, you should mention this to your doctor. He or she may ask you to stop this medication for a brief defined period of time (such as 2–4 weeks) and may perform a muscle blood test. If this brief discontinuation does not resolve the discomfort, then the original medication can almost always be safely restarted. If the muscle discomfort does indeed resolve when the statin medication is withdrawn, then you and your physician may still elect to restart the statin to be quite sure that the discomfort is related, or an alternative statin medication may be prescribed.

62. How can I quit smoking? When should I begin my efforts to quit smoking?

Smoking cessation is absolutely essential for all patients with PAD, and it is wisest to begin efforts to stop smoking immediately. When (not *if*) you succeed, you will be stopping the progression (worsening) of

PAD blockages, and you will markedly reduce your risk of developing new leg symptoms, worsened leg symptoms, or amputation. Ongoing tobacco use will make any other PAD treatment much less likely to work. You should not spend months or years "thinking about thinking about quitting," because the clock is ticking rapidly.

The most successful approach to achievement of complete tobacco cessation involves your recognition of the importance of ongoing tobacco use to your health, especially in the context of PAD, followed by an appointment with a nicotine or smoking dependency counselor. This individual will likely work with your doctor to offer a pharmacologic treatment to lower your addictive craving of tobacco (**Table 3**). All patients with PAD are encouraged to pick a specific "quit date" and to remove all cigarettes from their home. Prior to the quit date, a medication such as bupropion (Zyban) or varenacline (Chantix) may be prescribed to reduce the symptoms of nicotine withdrawal. Concomitant use of a prescribed or over-the-counter nicotine patch, gum, or inhaler may be useful as you plan your quit strategy.

63. How can I control high blood pressure?

Angiotensin-converting enzyme (ACE) inhibitor

A class of medications used for various therapeutic purposes, including to control high blood pressure, lower risk of future heart attack, or to preserve kidney function. This medication class is often recommended for individuals with PAD.

There are several classes of medications that effectively control high blood pressure for those with PAD. One class that is highly recommended is the **angiotensin-converting enzyme (ACE) inhibitor**. In past years, some physicians believed that a class of antihypertensive medications (beta blockers) might be prone to worsening claudication. This is a myth, and if your doctor believes you might benefit from use of a beta blocker medication, it is always appropriate to try. But, any medication or combination of medications that controls your blood pressure is appropriate.

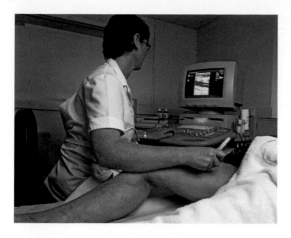

A. A patient undergoing a duplex arterial ultrasound test. (© Photo Researchers, Inc.)

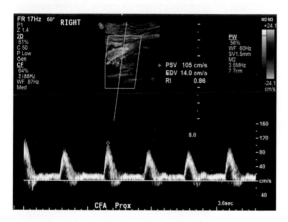

B. The test results from a duplex arterial ultrasound. These results show the dividing of the common femoral artery with no blockages in view.

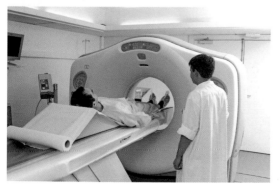

C. A patient undergoing a magnetic resonance (MR) angiogram test. (© Photo Researchers, Inc.)

D. A patient undergoing a computer tomography (CT) angiogram test. (© Photo Researchers, Inc.)

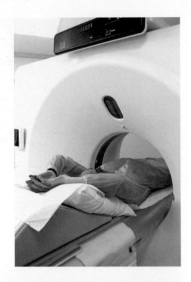

E. A CT angiogram test result showing stents in the common iliac arteries and superficial femoral arteries.

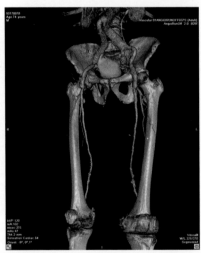

F. A patient undergoing a catheter-based angiogram test. (© Photo Researchers, Inc.)

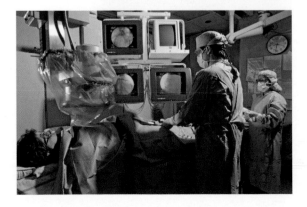

Table 3   Smoking and Peripheral Artery Disease

As an individual with vascular disease, you deserve access to key information that can improve your vascular health and that may save your life. You probably already are aware that tobacco use, in all of its forms, is damaging to your general health. We would like to share with you the following facts about tobacco and peripheral artery disease (PAD) to help you decide if you are willing to quit smoking.

- **Tobacco causes PAD** by increasing the formation of leg artery blockages, constricting blood vessels, and causing the blood to clot (with every puff).
- Tobacco is clearly the **most important cause of PAD**. Even a half pack of cigarettes per day may increase the risk of developing PAD by 30–50%.
- **Tobacco use causes heart attacks, strokes, and/or death** in as many as 5–15% of PAD patients per year. This means that as many as 50% of individuals with PAD who smoke **may develop one of these severe events within 5 years** after diagnosis.
- Tobacco causes PAD to progress much more rapidly, so that ≥ **1 in 5 patients** with claudication who smoke will develop leg pain at rest requiring a limb operation, such as artery bypass surgery, angioplasty, or amputation.
- Vascular surgery or angioplasty to repair blood vessels is **much less likely to be successful in patients who smoke**.
- **Amputation** is much more likely to occur in patients who smoke.
- Quitting smoking is associated with a **reduced risk of heart attack, stroke, and death rates** in patients with PAD.
- If you are thinking about quitting smoking, you should do so **as soon as possible**.

Unfortunately, few patients with PAD are told these important facts about tobacco use and PAD. We are committed to helping you stop smoking.

Source: Halverson SL, Hirsch AT. Tobacco and Peripheral Arterial Disease: Pathogenesis of PAD and the Management of Tobacco Addiction. In: *The Peripheral Arterial Disease Primary Care Series,* sponsored by the Society for Vascular Medicine and Biology, 1998-2000, a series of eight monographs on PAD care for office practice: Peripheral Arterial Disease and Risk Factor Management. Eds: Alan T. Hirsch, MD, Jonathan Halperin, MD.

64. How can I control diabetes?

Diabetes mellitus is the medical term for high blood sugar. The control of blood sugar involves lifestyle changes and drug treatment. The lifestyle change that most favorably impacts blood sugar level is weight loss.

The lifestyle change that most favorably impacts blood sugar level is weight loss.

In fact, medical studies indicate that significant weight loss may normalize blood sugar level. The initial treatment of diabetes is with pill forms of medication. If these medications do not control insulin effectively, then injection of insulin may be necessary.

65. How is prediabetes (metabolic syndrome) treated in order to reduce my chances of getting PAD and claudication?

The prediabetic state, or metabolic syndrome, most commonly occurs in obese individuals. Significant weight reduction can dramatically improve blood sugar levels, sometimes even into the normal range. A reduction in body fat is also accompanied by reduction in fat (triglycerides) in the bloodstream. A reduction in blood pressure may also occur with weight loss.

66. What type of diet lowers risk of PAD and reduces progression of PAD?

Although there are no long-term diet studies in patients with PAD, the scientific data indicate that a diet low in cholesterol will reduce the amount of cholesterol that sticks in artery plaque.

67. Does lowering homocysteine prevent or reduce plaque buildup in the arteries of the legs?

Homocysteine is a byproduct of protein breakdown. If elevated, it is associated with cholesterol buildup (plaque) in arteries, including those of the legs. See Question 48 for more on homocysteine. There are several published clinical studies indicating that lowering of homocysteine with folic acid and/or other B vitamins does not reduce the rate of heart attack or stroke.

There are no clinical studies that specifically evaluated the effect of homocysteine lowering on leg artery plaque. But given that this approach did not result in plaque stability in the heart arteries, it is extremely unlikely that homocysteine lowering has any impact on lower extremity arteries.

68. What is lipoprotein(a) and does it cause PAD?

Lipoprotein(a) is a type of cholesterol that circulates in the bloodstream and is associated with increased risk of heart attack and stroke. It is also associated with increased risk of developing PAD.

69. How are increased levels of lipoprotein(a) treated?

This type of cholesterol is difficult to lower, as it is not affected by diet, and blood levels are mostly determined by one's hereditary background. One medication, niacin, can lower blood lipoprotein(a) levels slightly, but there is no evidence that the use of niacin directly helps patients with PAD. One published study has indicated that lowering blood levels of the bad cholesterol (low-density lipoprotein, or LDL) decreases the adverse effects of elevated lipoprotein(a) and the associated increased risk of heart attack and stroke.

70. Can I prevent a heart attack or stroke by using aspirin or other antithrombotic (anticlotting) medications?

Yes, current medical guidelines highly recommend antiplatelet (also referred to as antithrombotic or anticlotting) medication for those with PAD. It is often asked why individuals with PAD do suffer such high rates of heart attack or stroke when the artery blockage

Lipoprotein(a)

A type of cholesterol that circulates in the bloodstream and is associated with increased risk of heart attack and stroke. It is also associated with increased risk of developing PAD.

Lowering Risk

is localized to the legs. In fact, these high rates exist even when heart or neck artery blockages are not severe and are not detected by standard cardiovascular stress tests. This risk is because even small amounts of coronary (heart) or carotid (neck) artery plaque can cause a clot to form that partially or fully obstructs the blood flow to the heart or brain tissue. When heart tissue dies from a lack of adequate blood flow, it is called a heart attack. When brain tissue dies from a lack of adequate blood flow, it is called a stroke.

Individuals with PAD benefit from use of aspirin, which prevents the formation of a clot when heart artery plaque ruptures.

Individuals with PAD benefit from use of aspirin, which prevents the formation of a clot when heart artery plaque ruptures. If aspirin cannot be used, an alternative medication called clopidogrel (Plavix) can accomplish a similar prevention of clot formation in the heart or brain arteries. Most physicians believe that both medications are similar in efficacy, although some data suggest that clopidogrel may be more effective in individuals with PAD. The choice of which of the two medications to use should be made with your doctor. There is no evidence that use of both medications together is more effective than one alone in individuals with PAD.

PART EIGHT

Noninvasive Treatment of Claudication

How does exercise improve walking?

How do I find a supervised exercise program?

Is there a pill for leg pain from PAD?

More . . .

There was a time when the only method to improve any of the leg symptoms associated with PAD was the performance of an "open" surgical operation, in which artery blockages were removed or bypassed by a vascular surgeon. Currently, individuals with PAD and claudication symptoms can enjoy benefit from any of four major treatment approaches, including use of supervised exercise, a claudication medication, angioplasty with or without stent placement, or open surgical procedures. An informed patient can now work with a physician to help select the best procedure, at the lowest risk, highest efficacy, and lowest cost, to maintain independence and lower the discomfort associated with claudication. Most individuals with PAD will never need a leg operation during their lifetime.

71. How do I improve painful walking (claudication)?

The first approach that should usually be tried for all patients who seek treatment of claudication involves use of exercise and pharmacologic treatment. Numerous studies have shown that a treadmill exercise program, preferably under medical supervision, improves walking ability. After 3 months of exercise training on a treadmill, patients can expect to double or even triple walking distance. There are no significant risks, and there are a tremendous number of other proven benefits.

72. How does exercise improve walking?

The exact mechanism(s) whereby exercise improves pain-free walking is unclear, but there is a well-founded scientific basis for this improvement, which involves several beneficial mechanisms. First, exercise has a direct effect on strengthening the leg muscles. By the time most individuals with PAD and claudication seek treatment, their leg muscles are profoundly deconditioned, meaning the muscles have atrophied and the remaining muscle is weak. Second, a program of exercise can increase the strength and endurance of muscle by directly improving the muscle metabolism. Third, exercise improves the connections between the nerves, which make the muscles contract, and the muscles themselves. Fourth, exercise decreases the production of inflammatory chemicals that can further hurt muscle and blood vessels. Fifth, and most critically, exercise improves endothelial function, which is the ability of the microscopic arterioles (the tiniest arteries) to relax and dilate and bring blood into the muscle. PAD is *not* merely a disease of large artery blockages. In PAD, the entire limb, including the microscopic blood vessels, nerves, and leg muscles are injured. A program of supervised exercise has been demonstrated to improve each of these injuries and improve walking. There are some clinical data to suggest that exercise may increase the size and number of blood vessels in the leg.

Exercise, when performed two to three times per week for a minimum of three months, is well established in helping patients double or triple their pain-free walking. This benefit is obtained when individuals participate in a supervised program. These results cannot be anticipated from casual home walking, as often results when a physician states, "Go home and walk." While this is good advice, it cannot substitute for a well-crafted professional program.

PAD is not merely a disease of large artery blockages. In PAD, the entire limb, including the microscopic blood vessels, nerves, and leg muscles are injured.

73. How do I find a supervised exercise program?

The truth is hard to fathom. Even though current scientific data and experience demonstrate that supervised exercise for claudication is safe, effective, and cost-effective, and that it is likely equal in efficacy to surgical and angioplasty treatments, it can be almost impossible to find a program to offer such care. This failure of access, widespread across the United States (but not so in other nations), is due to a combination of historic factors that led to barriers within Medicare and most other payers to provide reimbursement either to hospitals or to the patients who may be forced to pay directly for such treatment.

However, over the past few years, increasing numbers of insightful insurers and hospitals have begun to realize that there is almost no cost to them to add PAD exercise rehabilitation programs to their current cardiac rehabilitation programs. Therefore, practical steps you can take include:

1. Ask your doctor to write a formal referral to a PAD exercise program.
2. If your doctor does not know of a PAD-specific program in your area, ask for access to the largest available cardiac rehabilitation program, and discuss your needs with the program director. Most such directors understand the therapeutic power of PAD rehabilitation and will attempt to help you.
3. Discuss with your doctor and the rehabilitation director how payment might be made. There are choices: Your doctor can petition your healthcare insurer, the hospital can offer the care at discounted

rates, or you could choose to enroll as a "self-pay" patient.

If patients with PAD want equal access to proven and cost-effective therapies (the same as for patients with any disease), then they will have to demand this of their healthcare payers, government, and physicians.

74. Is there a pill for leg pain from PAD?

Yes, there are two medications approved by the Food and Drug Administration (FDA) for claudication in the United States—pentoxifylline (Trental) and cilostazol (Pletal). Of these, pentoxifylline is almost never used in the modern era, as its efficacy is extremely low. In one head-to-head study, patients taking cilostazol walked farther than those taking pentoxifylline. Of note, it usually takes at least 2 to 3 months before the beneficial effects of cilostazol are realized with improved pain-free walking.

Cilostazol does not reverse PAD, nor does it prevent heart attack and stroke. It *does* help individuals with claudication walk farther. It can be used safely in almost all patients with PAD and claudication. Some physicians believe that it works better in individuals with particular PAD anatomy (such as blockages farther down the leg). This is not true; the medication has equal efficacy in all patients with claudication, if it is going to work at all.

Cilostazol is now generic in the United States and is increasingly available throughout the world. In Europe and some other nations, other medications are also marketed to treat claudication. The efficacy of these other medications is not as well established.

75. Does cilostazol (Pletal) have side effects?

As with all medications, cilostazol has potential side effects, though it can be safely used in most individuals with claudication. The most common side effects of cilostazol are headache, palpitations (a feeling of extra heart beats), nausea, and loose bowel movements (or rarely diarrhea). These side effects are relatively infrequent and may disappear shortly after beginning the drug. If side effects occur, tell your doctor. The dosage of the medication may be adjusted or the medication may be briefly stopped to be sure that it was indeed this pill that caused the problem. Cilostazol should not be used in individuals with known heart failure. If you are unsure if this medication is appropriate for you, you simply need to ask your doctor.

76. Does cilostazol (Pletal) interact with other drugs?

Yes, several drugs cause higher blood levels of cilostazol that necessitate using the lower dose of 50 mg twice a day. These drugs may affect the removal of cilostazol from your system and include:

- Azole antifungals
- Macrolide antibiotics
- Diltiazem
- Nefazodone
- SSRI (selective serotonin reuptake inhibitor) antidepressants
- Cimetidine
- Rifamycins
- St. John's wort
- Certain antiseizure medications
- Esomeprazole
- Omeprazole

Blood thinners such as warfarin, aspirin, and clopidogrel can be safely used with cilostazol.

77. How do I prevent PAD and the leg artery blockages from worsening?

There are no therapies available to shrink plaque in the leg artery. The medical strategies employed aim at halting progression of plaque size and stabilizing the plaque that is present so that it does not rupture and cause a clot to develop. The mainstay of treatment is risk factor modification such as smoking cessation, reduction of cholesterol with statin drugs, control of blood pressure, and control of diabetes.

78. Are there experimental treatments for PAD?

Yes, there are several ongoing therapeutic strategies being tested for PAD. Novel treatments are generally grouped according to those aimed at improving claudication symptoms, those aimed at treating the plaque in the artery (to decrease rates of heart attack and stroke), and those aimed at treating critical limb ischemia (improving the chances of a skin ulcer healing or prevention of amputation).

79. What is therapeutic angiogenesis?

Therapeutic angiogenesis is a research (experimental and thus far unproven) strategy aimed at increasing the growth of arteries and capillaries in the body. For individuals with PAD, the goal of this approach is to improve the delivery of blood flow to the muscles or skin of the legs by increasing the number of smaller arteries. This treatment is only available in research studies.

Therapeutic angiogenesis

An experimental research strategy aimed at increasing the growth of arteries and capillaries in the body. For individuals with PAD, the goal of this approach is to improve the delivery of blood flow to the muscles or skin of the legs by increasing the number of smaller arteries.

Noninvasive Treatment of Claudication

Cell-based therapy

This is an experimental treatment that involves inserting living cells (usually bone marrow or circulating stem cells) into damaged or diseased tissue. This therapy is hypothesized to help grow new blood vessels and is being tested as a potential new approach to improve leg blood flow for individuals with PAD.

80. What is cell-based therapy for PAD?

Cell-based therapy is another research (experimental and thus far unproven) strategy that will hopefully provide a new approach to improving leg blood flow for individuals with PAD. The repair and maintenance of the lining of blood vessels involve local cells and also likely cells that grow in the bone marrow and then circulate in the blood. It is hoped that delivery of an increased number of adult stem cells, or modified mature vascular cells, will lead to an increased number of arteries in the legs that can carry blood around the areas of blockage. It is hoped that this will therefore improve leg circulation. This treatment is only available in research studies.

81. Can alcohol affect claudication?

While alcohol, used at levels of 1–2 beverages per day, has been observed to provide some potential long-term reduction in risk of developing PAD, alcohol has no known therapeutic benefit for individuals with established PAD. Specifically, there are no data to suggest that use of alcohol, in moderation or at any level, will improve or adversely affect claudication symptoms. Alternatively, there are no data to suggest that alcohol ingestion can modify the progression of PAD.

There are no data to suggest that use of alcohol, in moderation or at any level, will improve or adversely affect claudication symptoms.

82. Does ginkgo biloba help claudication symptoms?

Several clinical studies have been completed to evaluate the impact of ginkgo biloba on claudication symptoms. The results have indicated a very modest (small) improvement in walking distance of 50 meters or less, which is a rather tiny effect. In our clinical experiences, we cannot recall any patient ever stating to us that his or her symptoms improved significantly with use of ginkgo. This over-the-counter herbal substance is not recommended for claudication symptoms. Of note, high levels of ingestion of ginkgo can increase risk of bleeding when used in combination with medications such as aspirin that prevent clots from forming in the bloodstream.

83. Does chelation improve claudication symptoms?

The concept of **chelation** is an old one, remains popular, and continues to attract attention from individuals with PAD who seek an alternative approach to improving their symptoms or who wish for a method to reverse their disease. Unfortunately, there are no data that demonstrate that this dream is real for individuals with PAD, but use of chelation involves cost, misdirected hope, and some risk.

Chelation involves intravenous administration of a chelating agent such as EDTA (an abbreviation of the chemical compound, ethylenediaminetetraacetic acid). Although this medication was once shown to be useful for treating heavy metal toxicity, EDTA use has been studied and has *not* been proven useful in improving claudication symptoms. One prospective clinical study compared intravenous infusion of EDTA to a placebo (bicarbonate) and did not show any improvement in walking distance. There are no data to show that it can improve critical limb ischemia. There are no data to show that it can reverse atherosclerosis or improve existing artery blockages. Thus, chelation is not recommended to treat any aspect of PAD. While we wish for simple solutions, the truth is that to date, such wishful solutions do not exist.

Chelation

The concept that ingestion or intravenous infusion of chemicals could remove abnormal deposits of calcium from artery walls, thus shrinking or eliminating blockages. There is no scientific evidence that this works. The procedure is expensive, has no proven role in the treatment of PAD or heart disease, and may be dangerous.

Aerobic walking is the most beneficial form of exercise to improve claudication symptoms.

84. Is leg weight lifting beneficial in reducing claudication symptoms?

Isometric exercise with weights is beneficial in maintaining muscle strength and tone but has not been shown to improve the maximal pain-free walking ability. Aerobic walking is the most beneficial form of exercise to improve claudication symptoms.

85. Does biking exercise improve claudication symptoms?

There are some data that indicate bicycling exercise and even hand-crank aerobic exercise somewhat improve claudication symptoms. However, the most beneficial exercise is walking to the point where claudication symptoms occur and then resting until symptoms disappear. One should then resume walking to gain more benefit.

Mary's comment:

I never spoke to my doctor about this when discussing exercise. My main form of exercise is the use of a recumbent bike, and I assumed this was as good as walking. I am surprised to find out that walking has better outcomes than biking for the reduction of claudication symptoms.

86. Are there things I should not do if I have claudication?

Most importantly, you should not become or remain sedentary. In other words, "keep moving." The body was built to move against gravity, and to maintain health, it is essential to engage in daily physical activity no matter how old you are.

87. *Are there things I should* **not** *do if I have critical limb ischemia?*

You should not soak your feet in warm water, as this does not improve circulation and may even cause skin damage and worsen an ulcer.

PART NINE

Invasive Treatment of Claudication

What is an angioplasty of the leg artery?

What is a stent of the leg artery, and when is it used?

Is there a surgical bypass procedure that can improve blood flow for my blocked leg artery?

More...

It is a modern miracle that individuals with symptomatic PAD can be treated with "minimally invasive" methods, in which an artery can sometimes be opened in a one-hour procedure, replacing what had once been a long and sometimes complex operation. When these procedures are possible, great benefit can be obtained.

Yet, these procedures are not for every patient with PAD. You may ask, "If there are blockages in my leg arteries, wouldn't it always be better to open these?" or "If my arteries could be opened, how long will they stay open?" This section will help explain the use, benefit, and risk of invasive procedures to treat PAD.

88. My doctor used the term "interventional treatment." What does this mean?

The term *interventional* generally means an invasive approach in which a thin tube (a catheter) is threaded through the skin in order to directly view and treat an artery blockage. This approach is also called minimally invasive (compared with open surgical operations). Also, you may hear the terms *percutaneous*, meaning "through the skin" or *endovascular*, meaning "within the blood vessel." Another interventional treatment is a surgical approach to care that involves the removal of plaque or use of one of your own veins or a plastic tube to bypass a blocked leg artery. Both endovascular and surgical treatments can sometimes provide huge improvements in symptoms and can save threatened legs.

We note that the term interventional has become a standard professional medical phrase to describe treatments that open your body via small (percutaneous and endovascular) or larger "open" operations. Since "interventional" also tends to sound like "treatment," you should be aware that exercise, medications, and other lifestyle treatments are always considered first line and must be used with any invasive therapy. Thus, all PAD treatments (medical, pharmacologic, endovascular, and surgical) are truly "interventional approaches" to treating PAD.

89. What is an angioplasty of the leg artery?

An angioplasty is a medical term used to describe the opening of a clogged artery with a balloon-tipped catheter. A catheter is a plastic tube that is inserted in the artery through the skin via a small needle. Prior to catheter insertion, the skin will be numbed with an anesthetic medication so that there is minimal to no pain. Angioplasty is most effective for shorter and more proximal (closer to the groin) artery blockages and is less successful and less durable at artery sites below the mid-thigh.

90. When might I need an angioplasty?

An angioplasty of a leg artery is usually considered as one possible treatment when an individual suffers severe lifestyle-limiting claudication symptoms that persist despite the use of noninvasive medical treatments such as exercise or medications. Angioplasty is very commonly used as a major treatment for individuals who suffer acute limb ischemia (such as from the sudden development of a blood clot) or critical limb ischemia (defined as the slow onset of severe foot pain, nonhealing ulcers, or gangrene).

Angioplasty is not the right treatment for everyone. You or a loved one may be a potential candidate for leg artery angioplasty if an appropriately sized artery is involved (very small arteries are not usually well-treated

The decision as to whether angioplasty is appropriate depends on your symptoms, your overall health, and your leg artery anatomy.

by this procedure) and if the artery blockage is not too long. As always, the decision as to whether angioplasty is appropriate depends on your symptoms, your overall health, and your leg artery anatomy. Because the dye (contrast medication) that is used to visualize the artery can also hurt kidney function, angioplasty is often not appropriate for individuals who have decreases in kidney function. Thus, as with all medical treatments, this decision is not yours alone, but requires physician judgment to determine if this procedure will be successful, long-lasting, and low risk.

91. What are potential complications of leg artery angioplasty?

The potential short-term complications of a leg artery angioplasty include the following:

* Bleeding or bruising at the site of the catheter insertion at the groin
* Infection and damage of the artery or vein in the groin
* An allergic response to the dye (which can be mild, such as a rash; more challenging, such as impaired breathing or dangerously lowered blood pressure; or, rarely, fatal)
* Damage to the kidneys from the dye (which is usually reversible in individuals with normal kidney function but may be irreversible in individuals with damaged kidneys before the procedure)

The long-term complications of this procedure can include scar tissue formation at the site of the procedure, leading to a restenosis (reblockage) of the artery at the site at which it was treated. This restenosis of the treated site is more common in smaller arteries and in individuals who smoke or have diabetes. You should ask your physician his or her opinion as to what the chances are of restenosis of your blockage over short (one-year) and longer (five-year) time frames. This answer will help you decide if the procedure is right for you.

92. What is a stent of the leg artery, and when is it used?

A stent is a metal mesh tube that is sometimes used to hold open an artery that has been opened by use of a balloon angioplasty procedure (**Figure 12**). Arteries are not truly "pipes"; rather, they are living tissue that can scar or contract over time. Further, an artery that is treated by angioplasty can tear slightly after the balloon is inflated, and the tear can contribute to early restenosis (reblockage) of the artery. The treating physician may decide to place a stent in order to improve the chances of the artery staying open in the short term (immediate treatment time frame) or long term (years).

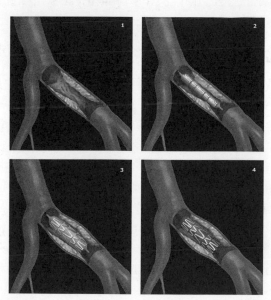

Figure 12 Placement of a balloon catheter (top two figures) and deployment of a stent in a leg artery (bottom two figures). (© Alexonline/ShutterStock, Inc.)

There are several types of stents manufactured from different types of metal and with different weaves of the metallic mesh. When such stents were created for treating heart artery blockages, physicians learned that covering the metal mesh with certain medications could also improve the chances of the artery staying open. The stent would be designed to slowly elute (meaning "leak") the medication to bathe the artery cells in the anti-growth medication. These drug-eluting stents have been proven to prevent restenosis in heart arteries. To date, none have proven to be useful in leg arteries.

93. What are potential complications of the leg artery stent?

The potential complications of the leg artery stent include restenosis (the slow reblockage of the artery within the stent) and clotting of the stent (which, rarely, occurs suddenly and usually soon after placement). Note that stents are used because restenosis of the affected artery when a stent is used is typically less frequent than when plain balloon angioplasty is used alone.

94. How long-lasting is treatment of a leg artery blockage by plain balloon angioplasty or by stent placement?

The amount of time that an artery stays open after angioplasty or stent placement depends on many factors. First, note that there is no permanent treatment of artery blockages, as the process that originally blocked the artery is usually still able to block arteries after angioplasty, stent placement, or surgical bypass. In other words, arteries are never "fixed"! One factor that affects the length of time an angioplasty or stent placement is effective is the severity of the original artery blockage prior to the procedure. Arteries with a short length of blockage also tend to do better over the long term than arteries with longer blockages. When the arteries beyond the blockage are more open, flow is faster and the angioplasty and/or stent placement also lasts longer. These are factors that you cannot affect. But, you *can* control important factors that are known to improve the durability of an angioplasty or stent placement. If you smoke, do not control your cholesterol, or do not take aspirin, the chances are greater that the treated artery segment will quickly reblock.

The restenosis rate after angioplasty of the iliac arteries near the groin is 20–40% over five years. The restenosis rate for the superficial femoral artery ranges from 30–50% over three years. For arteries below the knees (the anterior and posterior tibial arteries), as many as half of initially successfully treated blockages may reblock in as little as one year. Such quick reblockage may be reasonable to expect when one is trying to save a foot or leg from amputation in the short term. The reblockage rates may not be reasonable, however, for some patients with claudication in whom a more durable improvement is desired. Thus, overall, most patients should be aware of the success rates and limitations of angioplasty or stent placement at the site considered for treatment.

95. Is there a surgical bypass procedure that can improve blood flow for my blocked leg artery?

Yes, vascular surgical procedures also can be used to either open a blocked artery or to bypass the blockage to improve blood flow. These procedures are similar (usually longer) compared to bypasses performed on heart arteries (**Figure 13**). This surgical bypass is usually preferentially accomplished by use of one of a person's own leg veins. If a healthy leg vein is not available,

Invasive Treatment of Claudication

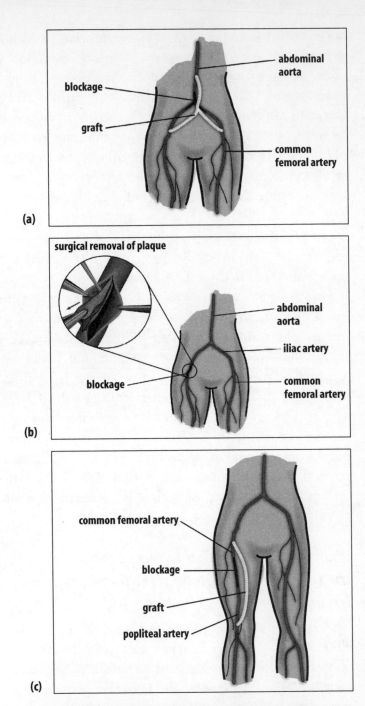

Figure 13 (a) Aorto-bifemoral bypass, (b) femoral artery endarterectomy, and (c) femoral–popliteal artery bypass.

a synthetic (plastic Dacron or Gore-Tex) graft or a preserved vein from a cadaver may be used for a bypass. The use of synthetic or cadaveric grafts may be very reasonable if critical limb ischemia is present or if the patient simply does not have a spare vein available. However, use of synthetic bypass graft is known to have a higher rate of reocclusion than when the bypass is performed using the patient's own natural vein.

96. What are potential complications of leg artery bypass?

The most common immediate complications from leg artery surgical bypass include bleeding and wound infection. Unfortunately, as for any direct procedure that opens a leg artery (similar to angioplasty), a leg artery bypass may also become blocked over time. Such reblocking is much more common in people who smoke, have diabetes, have uncontrolled high blood cholesterol, and/or do not take aspirin or other anti-clotting drugs.

For any surgical procedure on leg arteries, there is also a small risk of heart attack or stroke within the first 30 days after the procedure is completed. This risk may be as high as 2–5% within 30 days, or even higher if you smoke or have heart disease symptoms. Your doctor may not advise you to undertake an operative procedure if the risk to your heart is too high. Because of these concerns, both you and your doctor may prefer for you to undergo an angioplasty approach if this is feasible.

97. When should I have a surgical procedure to open up a leg artery?

The decision to undergo a procedure to open up a leg artery depends on the severity of your symptoms and the anatomy of your leg arteries (again, the length and severity of your artery blockages). For example, if you can walk three blocks without any significant pain in the muscles of your legs, then you may be able to improve adequately with other nonsurgical treatments. If so, it may be safest for you to defer any procedure unless your symptoms are extremely lifestyle limiting and if you have not benefited from a reasonable attempt to improve with alternative medical treatments.

Alternatively, if you have severe disease and symptoms of critical limb ischemia, then you are almost certainly a potential candidate for an urgent surgical or endovascular procedure to open up the artery. You should discuss with your vascular doctor the pros and cons of any procedure that is offered. Be informed regarding the name of the procedure, the potential benefits, the realistic risks to your leg and heart, as well as the anticipated length of time that the artery will stay open.

PART TEN

Your Doctor's Visit

What can I do to make my doctor's visit
as productive as possible?

How do I gain control over my life now that I have
PAD?

When you go to see either your primary care doctor or a vascular specialist, you can attend the visit prepared to better inform your doctor and to learn from your doctor. There may be real benefit in bringing a spouse, loved one, or friend to help support you during the visit. You may also want to bring a written record of your medical history and questions you would like answered.

98. What can I do to make my doctor's visit as productive as possible?

Before visiting your primary doctor or vascular specialist, you should try to remember the important details of your symptoms. Note when your leg symptoms first began. If your symptoms have changed since then, write down the date this change occurred. Note which leg is most bothersome. Do your symptoms limit your lifestyle? If so, exactly how? If you were better at the time your symptoms began, what activities would you then try to do that are difficult now? Regaining the ability to do the activities you "lost" can motivate both you and your physician.

Other questions you may want to prepare yourself to answer include:

- What leg is most affected?
- Which muscles or foot bother you and when?
- Do your legs hurt when you rest or sleep?
- Do your legs hurt when you stand for prolonged periods?
- If your legs hurt when you walk, at what distance does each leg begin to bother you?
- Are there any other illnesses that you know you have that also affect your legs?
- Have you ever had a wound that would heal slowly or not heal at all?

More technical medical questions may include:

- Do you know your risk factor numbers?
- What has been your personal record of blood pressures?
- Do you know your blood pressure goal, and have you reached it?
- Do you have copies of your blood cholesterol levels?

Make a list of all medications that you are taking and bring this list to the office. If this is difficult, bring the bottles of medication with you.

If your primary doctor has referred you to a specialist, which one was chosen and why? Does your doctor want the specialist to plan and offer overall treatment, or just one procedure? Will you be offered information on the alternative treatments that might also be effective?

Be prepared—just as you were for your primary care clinician—to review your vascular history in some detail. You may well want to bring a family member or friend with you to listen and take notes for you.

It is always helpful if you make a detailed list of all previous vascular or leg procedures you have had (whether on the neck, heart, or leg arteries). At which hospital were these procedures done and by what physician?

It would be most useful for the doctor to have a report and, if possible, images on a disk of any recent vascular studies that you may have completed (whether this was an ABI, stress test, ultrasound, or MR or CT angiogram). If you have seen other vascular specialists, try to obtain a copy of their consultation notes. If you have had prior operative or endovascular procedures, a copy of the operative or procedure notes can also be helpful.

Most vascular specialty offices will help obtain copies of all of these pieces of information on your behalf, but they can only seek the information if they know the basics of your history. You may benefit by writing this history into a log (perhaps on a computer, if one is available to you), and adding to this log as time goes by.

Knowing your own history and being able to share it with healthcare professionals will help you get the quality care you need.

Ideal PAD care is always lifelong. Knowing your own history and being able to share it with healthcare professionals will help you get the quality care you need.

When you leave the vascular specialty appointment, you usually should have heard a range of options for vascular care. These options may include different claudication treatments or different methods to improve CLI symptoms and outcomes. You should also have a definite plan to use an anticlotting medication (aspirin or clopidogrel), and have goals for the treatment of all risk factors.

99. How do I gain control over my life now that I have PAD?

Although PAD may have severely impaired your lifestyle, there are things that can be done to gain control over your life. These include modification of those risk factors that are in your control, such as smoking cessation, lowering cholesterol, and controlling blood pressure. You should know your own treatment targets and be responsible for achieving these specific goals.

If you are trying to improve your own walking, then recognize the importance of, and take responsibility for, having a very specific walking program in place. A supervised PAD exercise program is almost always superior to one that you might casually create on your own. Once you recognize that the discomfort itself—although somewhat painful—is not dangerous, you can be positive in your attitude that in the long run this program of exercise will give you back a better lifestyle and reduce your risk of heart attack and stroke.

Sometimes PAD is a result of actions that you took (choosing to smoke) or did not take (getting blood pressure or cholesterol checkups), so that you may wonder if you could have avoided having PAD. Guilt itself is not very helpful as you now try to improve and protect your life. Some people get PAD despite having made no mistakes regarding their risk factor control. Other people are fortunate in that they seem protected from developing PAD despite significant exposure to risk factors. Thus, do not dwell on the past. TAKE ACTION to control what you can. Stop smoking. Get to know PAD as an illness that you can survive, know that you usually have it in your power to improve, and forge a strong bond with your vascular clinician so that you can link your positive attitude to the physician's tools to get better.

Be willing to share your PAD diagnosis with friends and family. There is nothing embarrassing about having PAD, just as there is nothing embarrassing about having heart disease or any form of cancer. You deserve at least as much support from those who love you as any person with any illness. When you are able to share your fears, frustrations, hopes, and needs with others who love you, these individuals will be in a better position to help you.

If there are other members of your family, or friends, who are at risk for PAD (for example, children who smoke or who have elevated blood cholesterol), help them also take action to protect their health.

PART ELEVEN

Further Information on PAD

Where can I obtain further information
on PAD?

We hope that this book is helpful to you. We also hope that your own sense of hope is now so increased that you will actively seek answers to your ongoing questions, including many we may not have posed. Here are places to seek further information on PAD.

100. Where can I obtain further information on PAD?

You can read more about PAD and request information from the following organizations:

The Peripheral Arterial Disease (PAD) Coalition

The PAD Coalition unites efforts to improve the prevention, early detection, treatment, and rehabilitation of people with, or at risk for, PAD. It is an alliance of over 78 national leading health organizations, vascular health professional societies, and government agencies and corporations representing over 1 million health professionals working together to raise public and health professional awareness about PAD. It is a division of the Vascular Disease Foundation, a national nonprofit organization. The Coalition Web site includes patient education and information pages on PAD as well as clinical practice tools for health care providers (www.PADCoalition.org). It is your best source for PAD educational information.

The Vascular Disease Foundation

The Vascular Disease Foundation (VDF) is the leading national nonprofit organization that provides accurate and unbiased information on a full range of common vascular diseases. It is the Foundation's mission to improve health for all by reducing death and disability from vascular disease. The Vascular Disease Foundation leads efforts to educate the public and healthcare providers through awareness and education programs and through collaborations such as the PAD Coalition and the Venous Disease Coalition. Educational information provided includes an extensive patient-focused Web site, information pages, and a free quarterly newsletter, *Keeping in Circulation*, available online and in printed form. To join the Foundation's efforts, or for more information, please visit www.vdf.org or call 888.VDF.4INFO (888.833.4463).

The American Heart Association

The American Heart Association is guided by its mission to build healthier lives free of cardiovascular diseases and stroke. Information regarding atherosclerosis risk factors, PAD, stroke, and their treatment can be found at its Web site (www.hearthub.org).

National Heart, Lung, and Blood Institute

The National Heart, Lung, and Blood Institute (NHLBI) of the National Institutes of Health has created the "Stay in Circulation: Take Steps to Learn About P.A.D." national public awareness campaign. Free access to this information can be obtained at www.aboutpad.org.

Glossary

Acute arterial occlusion (or acute limb ischemia [ALI]): A sudden and complete occlusion (blockage) of an artery in the leg. This presentation of PAD is quite uncommon and is typically due to either a blood clot (thrombus) traveling from a site upstream, such as from the heart or the aortic artery, or from a popliteal artery aneurysm to a more distant leg artery.

Aneurysm: An expansion or "ballooning" of the aorta or other arteries. Not all aneurysms are dangerous, but all should be followed by your doctor to verify if they are expanding.

Angioplasty: A procedure that opens clogged arteries by compressing obstructing plaque against the artery wall by inflation of a small balloon that is on the tip of the catheter.

Angiotensin-converting enzyme (ACE) inhibitor: A class of medications used for various therapeutic purposes, including to control high blood pressure, lower risk of future heart attack, or to preserve kidney function. This medication class is often recommended for individuals with PAD.

Ankle-brachial index (ABI) test: A noninvasive, safe, and inexpensive blood pressure test that compares the higher (systolic) blood pressures that are recorded at the arms and ankles. This test is usually required for all individuals with PAD.

Aorta: The major artery that leaves the heart and whose branches supply the rest of the body.

Arterial entrapment syndrome: A rare condition where arteries (which must often travel between muscle groups, or between muscles and bones, in order to reach the arms and legs) become briefly blocked or "entrapped" during very vigorous exercise. This can sometimes be an unusual cause of claudication.

Arteries: Blood vessels that carry blood away from the heart, supplying nutrition and oxygen to all of the tissues of the body.

Aspirin: Acetylsalicylic acid, or ASA, is a non-prescription, anti-inflammatory medication that is used to reduce pain and fever. This medication is also proven to prevent blood from clotting in the arteries, and thus lowers the risk of heart attack or stroke in individuals who are at risk.

Atherosclerosis: A blockage of the inner lining of an artery by cholesterol deposits, resulting in poor blood flow to the skin, muscles, or other body organs. This disease, also known as "hardening of the arteries," is caused by smoking, diabetes, high blood pressure, elevated blood cholesterol, or inherited factors. Atherosclerosis is the most common cause of lower extremity PAD.

Beta blockers (β-blockers): A class of antihypertensive medications that lower blood pressure and lower the risk of heart attack.

Catheter: A small flexible plastic tube that is inserted through the skin into an artery or vein and then used to inject solutions into the blood stream. The procedure used to place a catheter into the body is called a "catheterization."

Catheter angiogram: An invasive test that uses special tubes (catheters) that are passed through the skin, usually from the groin, into the arteries. A solution that is opaque on X-Rays (a "dye") is then injected through the tube into the arteries so they appear clearly on an X-ray. An angiogram usually takes approximately one hour.

Cell-based therapy: This is an experimental treatment that involves inserting living cells (usually bone marrow or circulating stem cells) into damaged or diseased tissue. This therapy is hypothesized to help grow new blood vessels and is being tested as a potential new approach to improve leg blood flow for individuals with PAD.

Chelation: The concept that ingestion or intravenous infusion of chemicals could remove abnormal deposits of calcium from artery walls, thus shrinking or eliminating blockages. There is no scientific evidence that this works. The procedure is expensive, has no proven role in the treatment of PAD or heart disease, and may be dangerous.

Claudication: Fatigue, discomfort, or pain that occurs in the leg muscles during exercise and that always resolves promptly with rest. This symptom usually occurs reproducibly at the same walking distance day-to-day, and can be considered as "angina of the legs." Claudication is a common symptom of PAD and results from blockages in the arteries that prevent blood, oxygen, and nutrients from reaching the working muscles.

Computerized tomographic (CT) angiogram: A noninvasive method of looking at arteries inside the body using a donut shaped X-ray camera and intravenous dye. Two- and three-dimensional, highly detailed images of arteries are possible with this method.

Coronary arteries: The arteries that supply blood, oxygen, and nutrients to the heart.

Coronary heart disease: Heart disease caused when the arteries that supply the heart are narrowed by plaque buildup, which can lead to both angina and heart attack.

Critical limb ischemia (CLI): One of the most severe manifestations of PAD in which the blood flow to the legs and feet is decreased to the point where there is pain, even at rest, wounds do not heal promptly, and tissue death (or "gangrene") occurs. Without prompt treatment, amputation may be necessary.

Deep vein thrombosis (DVT): A blood clot in the deep veins of the leg. This disease is not related to PAD.

Diabetes: A condition where the body is unable to produce or use insulin properly, causing too high levels of sugar in the blood. Diabetes is one of the major risk factors for PAD.

Duplex arterial ultrasound: A noninvasive test that uses sound waves (ultrasound) to measure how blood moves through arteries and that can define the presence of artery blockages without exposure to X-rays.

Embolism: The condition that occurs when a blood clot travels from the heart to a more distant artery, blocking flow of blood.

Fibromuscular dysplasia: A condition, also known as FMD, caused when there is abnormal growth of the artery walls, which can cause a decrease in blood flow. When this occurs in the neck (carotid or verte-bral) arteries, a stroke may occur. When this occurs in the arteries to the kidneys, hypertension may occur.

Gangrene: When tissue dies due to lack of blood flow. Gangrene is a sign of severe PAD, and if blood flow is not improved immediately, amputation may be required.

Heart stress test: A test designed to measure if there are severe heart (coronary) artery blockages. Such a stress test can be performed using either treadmill or bicycle exercise, or using medications that increase heart rate and heart function, instead of exercise, for individuals with PAD who may not be able to walk or run vigorously.

High-sensitivity C-reactive protein (hs-CRP): A protein that exists in the blood of all people and that increases in response to infection or inflammatory diseases (like some arthritis conditions). It is also increased in individuals with progressive atherosclerosis.

Homocysteine: A natural amino acid in the body that is needed to maintain good health. Too high levels in the blood, however, can damage artery walls or cause blood clots, and may be a risk factor for developing PAD. There is no evidence that treating elevated homocysteine levels has any beneficial therapeutic effect.

Large vessel arteritis: Rather rarely, arteries can be damaged by diseases that cause inflammation of the artery wall. These diseases are treated very differently than when arteries are affected by atherosclerosis.

Lipoprotein(a): A type of cholesterol that circulates in the bloodstream and is associated with increased risk of heart attack and stroke. It is also associated with increased risk of developing PAD.

Lymphatics: Microscopic vessels that transport fluid and protein from all of the tissues of the body, and that connect to the lymph glands. When these tiny vessels are blocked, swelling can occur that is called "lymphedema." This disease has no relationship to PAD.

Lymphedema: Leg swelling caused by blockages in the small lymphatic blood vessels.

Magnetic resonance (MR) angiogram: A noninvasive method of looking at arteries inside the body using MR imaging. The body is passed into a long tube and an intravenous medication is injected to permit the arteries to be visible.

Metabolic syndrome: A high-risk condition in which a group of multiple risk factors coexist. These risk factors include an elevated blood sugar near the diabetic range, low good cholesterol (HDL), high triglyceride levels, and high blood pressure. The underlying problem is an inability of insulin (the hormone secreted from the pancreas that controls blood sugar) to work properly. Metabolic syndrome increases the risk of development of PAD.

Peripheral artery disease (PAD): The broad group of disorders that affect any artery other than those that supply the heart itself. In most common usage, PAD implies disease of the arteries that supply the legs, as most recognized illness occurs in these vessels.

Phlegmasia cerulea dolens: A rare condition where DVT blockage of blood *out* of the leg impairs the heart's ability to pump blood *into* the leg. When this occurs, the blood flow to the leg arteries may cause muscle pain even at rest.

Plaque: Fatty deposits that narrow or clog arteries and can cause PAD.

Popliteal adventitial cysts: The popliteal artery can in rare cases be blocked by "cystic adventitial disease." These cysts develop between the middle and outer layers of the wall of this knee artery. The cause of these cysts is unknown, could be hereditary or due to repetitive artery trauma. Such cysts occur more frequently in young men with new onset of claudication.

Radiopaque dye: The dye injected into arteries during an angiogram to permit X-rays to provide a detailed picture of their size and direction.

Restenosis: A recurring narrowing of an artery after any corrective treatment such as angioplasty or bypass surgery.

Statin: A class of cholesterol-lowering drugs that is best proven to lower rates of heart attack, stroke, or death.

Stent: A tubular metal device that is implanted into a blocked artery to hold it open and allow freer flow of blood.

Therapeutic angiogenesis: An experimental research strategy aimed at increasing the growth of arteries and capillaries in the body. For individuals with PAD, the goal of this approach is to improve the delivery of blood flow to the muscles or skin of the legs by increasing the number of smaller arteries.

Thromboangiitis obliterans: A relatively rare disease, also called Buerger's disease, that is associated with inflammation and clotting of the arteries beyond the elbows and knees. It is more common in young men who use tobacco, though its cause is unknown.

Thrombosis: The condition that occurs when blood clots develop in an artery.

Toe-brachial index: A test that is used to diagnose PAD that is performed by measuring the relative blood pressures in the great toes and arms. This test is especially useful in individuals with diabetes and those in whom the ABI test is not accurate.

Transcutaneous oximetry ($TcPO_2$) test: A test that uses oxygen-sensing electrodes to measure the delivery of oxygen to the skin tissue. This test is used often in individuals with slow-healing skin wounds.

Ulcer: The loss of a layer of skin tissue, due to injury, infection, damaged sensory nerves, or PAD. Skin ulcers, regardless of cause, are most dangerous in the presence of any severe impairment of blood flow, as occurs in some individuals with PAD.

Veins: Blood vessels that return blood from body tissue back to the heart.

Venous insufficiency: A medical problem that occurs when leg veins are unable to function efficiently due to prior blockage or to the presence of leaky vein valves that impair the rapid return of blood to the heart.

Index